New Treatments for Chemical Addictions

Review of Psychiatry Series

John M. Oldham, M.D., and
Michelle B. Riba, M.D., Series Editors

New Treatments for Chemical Addictions

EDITED BY
Elinore F. McCance-Katz, M.D., Ph.D.,
and
Thomas R. Kosten, M.D.

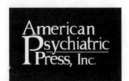

American Psychiatric Press, Inc.

Washington, DC
London, England

Note: The authors have worked to ensure that all information in this book concerning drug dosages, schedules, and routes of administration is accurate as of the time of publication and consistent with standards set by the U.S. Food and Drug Administration and the general medical community. As medical research and practice advance, however, therapeutic standards may change. For this reason and because human and mechanical errors sometimes occur, we recommend that readers follow the advice of a physician who is directly involved in their care or the care of a member of their family.

Copyright © 1998 American Psychiatric Press, Inc.

01 00 99 98   4 3 2 1
First Edition
ALL RIGHTS RESERVED

Manufactured in the United States of America on acid-free paper

American Psychiatric Press, Inc.
1400 K Street, N.W.
Washington, DC, 20005
www.appi.org

Library of Congress Cataloging-in-Publication Data
New treatments for chemical addictions / edited by Elinore F.
McCance-Katz and Thomas R. Kosten.
　　p.　　cm. —. (Review of psychiatry series, ISSN 1041-5882)
　　Includes bibliographical references and index.
　　ISBN 0-88048-838-7
　　1. Drug abuse. 2. Dual diagnosis. 3. Alcoholism—Sex factors.
　I. Kosten, Thomas R.　II. Series.
　　[DNLM: 1. Diagnosis, Dual (Psychiatry). 2. Tobacco Use Disorder—
diagnosis. 3. Alcohol-Related Disorders—diagnosis. 4. Opioid-
Related Disorders—diagnosis. 5. Substance-Related Disorders—
therapy. 6. Psychotherapy—methods. WM 270 A2243 1998]
　　RC564.A2914　1998
　　616.86—dc21
　　DNLM/DLC
　　for Library of Congress　　　　　　　　　　　　　　　　98-6546
　　　　　　　　　　　　　　　　　　　　　　　　　　　　　　CIP

British Library Cataloguing in Publication Data
A CIP record is available from the British Library.

Contents

Contributors

Robert Paul Cabaj, M.D.   Medical Director, San Mateo Mental Health Services; and Associate Clinical Professor in Psychiatry, University of California, San Francisco

H. Westley Clark, M.D., J.D., M.P.H.   Associate Clinical Professor of Psychiatry, University of California, San Francisco; and Chief, Associated Substance Abuse Programs, San Francisco Veterans Affairs Medical Center

Tony P. George, M.D.   Neuropsychopharmacology Fellow, Yale University School of Medicine, Department of Psychiatry, New Haven, Connecticut

Thomas R. Kosten, M.D.   Chief of Psychiatry, VA Connecticut; and Professor, Yale University School of Medicine, Department of Psychiatry, New Haven, Connecticut

Elinore F. McCance-Katz, M.D., Ph.D.   Director, Yale Medications Development Research Center; and Assistant Professor, Yale University School of Medicine, Department of Psychiatry, New Haven, Connecticut

Terry Michael McClanahan, M.A.   Doctoral student, Department of Counseling Psychology, University of San Francisco; and Public Policy Analyst, University of California, San Francisco

John M. Oldham, M.D.   Director, New York State Psychiatric Institute; and Professor and Vice Chairman, Department of Psychiatry, Columbia University College of Physicians and Surgeons, New York, New York

Michelle B. Riba, M.D.   Clinical Associate Professor of Psychiatry and Associate Chair for Education and Academic Affairs, Department of Psychiatry, University of Michigan Health System, Ann Arbor, Michigan

Myroslava K. Romach, M.Sc., M.D., F.R.C.P.C. Assistant Professor, Psychopharmacology and Dependence Research Unit, Women's College Hospital; Centre for Research in Women's Health and Department of Psychiatry, University of Toronto, Toronto, Canada

Edward M. Sellers, M.D., Ph.D., F.R.C.P.C. Professor, Psychopharmacology and Dependence Research Unit, Women's College Hospital; Centre for Research in Women's Health and Departments of Pharmacology, Medicine and Psychiatry, University of Toronto, Toronto, Canada

Susan M. Stine, M.D., Ph.D. Director, Opiate Treatment Program, and Assistant Professor of Psychiatry, Yale University, VA Connecticut Healthcare System, West Haven, Connecticut

Stephen A. Wyatt, D.O. Addiction Psychiatry Fellow, Yale University School of Medicine, Department of Psychiatry, New Haven, Connecticut

Douglas M. Ziedonis, M.D., M.P.H. Associate Professor, Yale University School of Medicine, Department of Psychiatry, New Haven, Connecticut

Introduction to the Review of Psychiatry Series

John M. Oldham, M.D., and Michelle B. Riba, M.D.,
Series Editors

Beginning with 1998, the annual Review of Psychiatry adopts a new format. What were individual sections bound together in a large volume will be published only as independent monographs. Each monograph provides an update on a particular topic. Readers may then selectively purchase those monographs of particular interest to them. Last year, Volume 16 was available in the large volume and individual monographs, and the individually published sections were immensely successful. We think this new format adds flexibility and convenience to the always popular series.

Our goal is to maintain the overall mission of this series—that is, to provide useful and current clinical information, linked to new research evidence. For 1998 we have selected topics that overlap and relate to each other: 1) Psychopathology and Violent Crime, 2) Addictions, 3) Psychological Trauma, 4) Psychobiology of Personality Disorders, 5) Child Psychopharmacology, and 6) Interpersonal Psychotherapy. All of the editors and chapter authors are experts in their fields. The monographs capture the current state of knowledge and practice while providing guideposts to future lines of investigation.

We are indebted to Helen ("Sam") McGowan for her dedication and skill and to Linda Gacioch for all of her help. We are indebted to the American Psychiatric Press, Inc., under the leadership of Carol C. Nadelson, M.D., who has supported this important and valued review series. We thank Claire Reinburg, Pamela Harley, Ron McMillen, and the APPI staff for all their generous assistance.

Foreword

Elinore F. McCance-Katz, M.D., Ph.D., and
Thomas R. Kosten, M.D.

Drug and alcohol abuse are an enduring problem in the United States. The public health implications of this tremendous problem are alarming. Substance abuse accounts for a large percentage of health care dollars spent in this country as a result of treating the acute and chronic medical conditions and mental disorders directly attributable to drug and alcohol abuse. Substance abuse also permeates and contributes to many of the social problems we face in this nation today, including crime, violence in the family, child abuse and neglect, poverty, lack of education and attainment of work skills, and loss of workplace productivity. As a society, we all pay the costs of substance abuse, either directly or indirectly.

In 1995 an estimated 12.8 million Americans (6.1% of the population age 12 or older) were current users of illegal drugs (National Institute on Drug Abuse [NIDA] 1996). Although this number has been fairly stable since 1992, data collected on the use of cigarettes shows increasing use among young people since 1991. Current rates of cigarette smoking are more than 9% in 8th graders, more than 16% in 10th graders, and nearly 22% in 12th graders. About 61 million Americans (29% of the population over age 12) are smokers. Although there is no predominance of smoking by race or ethnicity in the United States, smoking is correlated negatively with educational status. Smokers are more likely to be heavy drinkers and users of illegal drugs. Likewise for alcohol, approximately 111 million Americans older than 12 years report alcohol use; 11 million of these are heavy drinkers and are more likely to be illicit drug users.

Given these data, it is especially timely to devote a *Review of*

This chapter was supported by Grants K-20-DA (E.F.M.) and X02 (T.R.K.) from the National Institute on Drug Abuse.

Psychiatry monograph to topics in addiction psychiatry. Every practicing psychiatrist must struggle with issues of addiction and its related medical, psychological, and social problems in the treatment of the mentally ill. Yet residency training has only recently begun to systematically address the treatment of patients with substance-related disorders. Therefore, in this monograph, selected important topics have been addressed by experts in the field.

The widespread problem of nicotine dependence, which is conferred primarily through cigarette smoking, is one in which considerable strides have been made in understanding the neurobiology of nicotine, the contribution of nicotine to psychiatric and other substance-related disorders and their treatment, and the development of effective pharmacotherapies. In Chapter 1, "Current Issues in Nicotine Dependence and Treatment," Ziedonis et al. review recent guidelines from the American Psychiatric Association on the treatment of nicotine dependence (American Psychiatric Association 1996), including assessment, treatment, comorbidity, and prevention. The critical role of psychiatrists in the treatment of nicotine dependence is directly related to the high prevalence of comorbid nicotine dependence among depressed and psychotic patients. Pharmacotherapies can be integrated with behavioral management techniques that are individualized to the needs of the patient, whether he or she is a person with a single diagnosis of nicotine dependence, a dually diagnosed patient with a psychiatric disorder in addition to nicotine dependence, or a triply diagnosed patient—one with nicotine dependence, other substance-related disorders, and mental illness.

Basic science and treatment research for alcohol-related disorders has been overwhelmingly conducted in men, despite epidemiological data showing that as many as 10.7 million American women may use alcohol abusively (Center for Substance Abuse Treatment 1994). Over the past few years, research has begun to identify differences between men and women who use alcohol. Frezza et al. (1990) have reported on higher blood ethanol concentrations in women relative to men after accounting for differences in size. It has been shown that women have lower activity of gastric alcohol dehydrogenase, resulting in less first-pass metabolism of ingested alcohol and constituting a significant mechanism by which higher alcohol levels are obtained in women. This has been shown to enhance the vulnerability of women to acute and chronic complications of alcoholism. In addition, total body water of women is, on average, less than that of men, which may also contribute to higher alcohol concentrations in women (Marshall et al. 1983). These findings suggest an explanation for the significantly shorter interval between the age at which women first begin to experience alcohol-related problems and then seek treatment (Piazza et al. 1989).

These findings underscore the basis for Chapter 2, "Alcohol Dependence: Women, Biology, and Pharmacotherapy," by Romach and Sellers on women and alcohol. They review the epidemiology and natural history of alcohol use in women, metabolic and kinetic differences between men and women, and the consequences of alcohol abuse in women. This comprehensive review reports on the effects of alcohol in women, taking into account the effects of female hormonal status and menstrual cycle as well as the contribution of oral contraceptive and hormonal replacement treatment in alcohol pharmacokinetics and pharmacodynamics. The authors also relate alcohol use to comorbid psychiatric disorders and provide a discussion of women's responses to alcoholism treatment. This chapter is of particular relevance to any clinician seeing psychiatric or substance abuse patients.

The National Household Survey on Drug Abuse (Substance Abuse and Mental Health Services Administration 1995) estimates that 2 million people have used heroin at least once. Furthermore, NIDA estimates that there are more than 500,000 heroin-addicted people in the United States, about 115,000 of whom are being treated in 750 methadone maintenance programs located in 40 states (Center for Substance Abuse Treatment 1993). It is clear that many more addicted individuals are in need of treatment than are currently receiving it. To address the problem of treatment availability, clinical research in recent years has significantly expanded the repertoire of available treatments for this population. This increased availability of treatment slots has also expanded the variety of settings in which to receive treatment for opioid dependence. In Chapter 3, "Opiate Dependence and Current Treatments," Stine provides a comprehensive overview of currently available and soon-to-be available opioid maintenance treatments for these patients, including standard methadone maintenance treatment; *l*-α-acetylmethadol (LAAM), a long-acting, methadone-like drug; and buprenorphine, an opioid with both agonist and antagonist properties. The issue of comorbid substance abuse in opioid-dependent patients and treatment strategies directed toward this comorbidity are reviewed for the practicing clinician. The difficulty in engaging women who are opioid dependent in currently available treatment programs is reviewed, as are the factors that contribute to the difficulty in engaging opioid-dependent females in treatment. Pregnant opioid-dependent women represent a particularly challenging subpopulation needing coordination of care among several medical specialties and systems. Other special populations who require specialized treatment and coordination of care include those with severe medical illnesses such as liver disease or HIV disease. This chapter also reviews how to optimally manage medically ill, opioid-maintained patients who often receive multiple medications that may have pharmacokinetic interactions with methadone.

Illicit drug use is inextricably linked to the spread of infectious diseases such as HIV disease and AIDS. Injection drug use has become the leading risk factor for new HIV infection in the United States. Approximately 30% of new AIDS cases reported through June 1996 were related to sharing of contaminated needles, heterosexual contact with an infected injection drug user, or maternal injection of illegal drugs (NIDA 1996). Crack cocaine smokers, particularly women who trade sex for drugs, are also at high risk for HIV infection: Prevalence rates among these women are as high as 30% in some communities. The risk of HIV infection is also increased when unsafe sex occurs often under the influence of drugs or alcohol.

These statistics underscore the importance of understanding the relationship between HIV disease and substance abuse, a topic covered thoroughly in Chapter 4, "Substance Abuse and HIV Diseases: Entwined and Intimate Entities," by Cabaj. This chapter overviews the epidemiology and enmeshment of HIV and substance abuse. Critically important to effective treatment of this population is an understanding of the process of medical and psychiatric evaluation and management. The clinician is given the essential information needed to initiate and maintain the treatment relationship and suggestions on how to effect behavioral change in the substance abuser with HIV disease. Multiple losses are experienced by these patients, including that of health, loved ones, and financial security. Psychiatric illness, particularly depression and anxiety, is common in the substance abuser with HIV disease. A discussion of the treatment of psychiatric disorders and psychopharmacology in this population provides a framework in which to consider the needs of these triply diagnosed patients. Special attention is paid to issues that occur with unfortunate frequency in the substance abuser with HIV disease, particularly suicidality and its assessment and treatment.

In recent years, mental health professionals have become increasingly aware of dual diagnosis, the comorbid occurrence of substance-related and psychiatric disorders. Specialized inpatient and intensive outpatient or partial hospital programs have been developed to provide for the needs of the severely ill dually diagnosed patient, but these resources are limited and often serve only the most severely ill patients. In their review in Chapter 5, "Contemporary Issues in Dual Diagnosis," Clark and McClanahan point out that the mental health treatment system remains, for the most part, dichotomized—that is, in usual practice, psychiatric disorders are treated in the mental health system and substance abuse is treated in clinics specializing in drug and alcohol abuse treatment. As the authors discuss, this dichotomized system works to the detriment of many patients who are dually diagnosed but remain unidentified as such because of the lack of expertise in each system for recognition of the comorbid disorder(s) and provision of integrated treatment. The authors underscore the importance of recognizing substance abuse in psychiatric patients by mental health care providers and emphasize that nearly all psychiatric symptoms reported by patients can be consistent with substance-induced effects. There are high rates of comorbidity: 47% of all individuals with a lifetime diagnosis of schizophreniform disorders or schizophrenia, 24% of those with an anxiety disorder, 32% of those with any affective disorder, and 61% of those with bipolar I disorder have a comorbid substance use disorder (Regier et al. 1990). Thus, it is crucial for clinicians to obtain a substance use history from all patients, and confirmatory testing (urine toxicology screens or Breathalyzer tests) should be used therapeutically.

Clark and McClanahan go on to discuss the process of diagnostic evaluation and to review an important but little-reviewed area in the literature—that of legal issues surrounding treatment of patients with substance-related disorders. Issues of pharmacotherapy in dually diagnosed patients are discussed in detail to help clinicians select specific psychotropic medications and to be aware of the pros and cons of particular medications. Clinicians will find this information helpful in the day-to-day treatment of these challenging patients. Several special diagnostic issues in dual diagnosis are discussed briefly, including sexual abuse, eating disorders, and combat-related posttraumatic stress disorder. Finally, the authors provide a framework for integrating therapies and addressing the needs of staff members in order to provide optimal treatment to these complex patients. The authors point out that in dually diagnosed patients, treatment of only the psychiatric disorder will not effectively treat the substance abuse, and treatment of substance abuse alone in patients with active psychiatric disorders places such patients at high risk for relapse to substance abuse. In these multiple ways, this chapter will aid the clinician in treating the dually diagnosed patient.

References

American Psychiatric Association: Practice guideline for the treatment of patients with nicotine dependence. Am J Psychiatry 153(suppl): 1–31, 1996

Center for Substance Abuse Treatment: State methadone treatment guidelines. Treatment Improvement Protocol No 1. Rockville, MD, Center for Substance Abuse Treatment, 1993

Center for Substance Abuse Treatment: Practical Approaches in the Treatment of Women Who Abuse Alcohol and Other Drugs. Rockville, MD, Center for Substance Abuse Treatment, 1994

National Institute on Drug Abuse: Drug abuse and drug abuse research: the fifth triennial report to Congress from the Secretary, Department of Health and Human Services. Bethesda, MD, National Institute on Drug Abuse, November 1996

Frezza M, Di Padova C, Pozzato G, et al: High blood alcohol levels in women: the role of decreased gastric alcohol dehydrogenase activity and first-pass metabolism. N Engl J Med 322:95–99, 1990

Marshall AW, Kingstone D, Boss M, et al: Ethanol elimination in males and females: relationship to menstrual cycle and body composition. Hepatology 3:701–706, 1983

Piazza NJ, Vrbka JL, Yeager RD: Telescoping of alcoholism in women alcoholics. Int J Addict 24:19–28, 1989

Regier DA, Framer ME, Rae DS, et al: Comorbidity of mental disorders with alcohol and other drug abuse: results from the Epidemiologic Catchment Area (ECA) study. JAMA 264:2511–2518, 1990

Substance Abuse and Mental Health Services Administration, Office of Applied Studies: Preliminary estimates from the 1994 National Household Survey on Drug Abuse. Advance Report No 10. Rockville, MD, Substance Abuse and Mental Health Services Administration, 1995

Chapter 1

Current Issues in Nicotine Dependence and Treatment

Douglas M. Ziedonis, M.D., M.P.H.,
Stephen A. Wyatt, D.O., and Tony P. George, M.D.

This is an important time for mental health clinicians to be knowledgeable about the risks and costs of smoking and to encourage their patients to quit smoking. Indeed, this is an exciting time to be working in the field of tobacco addiction; major changes in public policy and public opinion are strongly in favor of helping individuals to quit smoking and of educating at-risk populations, particularly teenagers, about the dangers of tobacco use. Ongoing advances in research are helping us to better understand the basic mechanisms of nicotine dependence and are leading to an array of new clinical treatment approaches, including pharmacotherapy advances of nicotine replacement (spray, inhaler, over-the-counter patch and gum), bupropion (Zyban), and new combinations of medications (multiple patches, patch and gum, bupropion and patch, etc.). In this review, we summarize the important assessment and treatment issues for nicotine addiction, focusing on the smoker with coexisting psychiatric and/or substance abuse problems.

The authors thank Drs. John R. Hughes, Jack E. Henningfield, and Serdar Dursun for their careful review and helpful comments. Supported by Grants K20-DA00193 (D.M.Z.), P50-DA09241 (B.J.R.), and RO1-DA09127 (D.M.Z.) from the National Institute on Drug Abuse (NIDA); a NIDA Addictions Research Fellowship (T32 DA-07238, for S.A.W.); a Physician-Scientist Fellowship Award from the L. P. Markey Foundation; and a Young Investigator Award from National Alliance for Research on Schizophrenia and Depression (NARSAD) (T.P.G.).

Why should psychiatrists and mental health specialists be interested in this topic? As a profession, we value a holistic approach to patient care in which biopsychosocial issues are considered. Most of our patients smoke, and they are at high risk for death from smoking-related illnesses. Current chronic smokers have higher rates of psychiatric comorbidity and of other substance use disorders, more severe nicotine dependence, and lower motivation to quit smoking.

Tobacco addiction, like other forms of addiction, remains a common problem in the general population and in the mental health setting. It has enormous health consequences. Tobacco use is the chief avoidable cause of morbidity and mortality in our society: More than 400,000 deaths are attributed to cigarette smoking each year. Smoking is a known cause of cancer, heart disease, stroke, and chronic obstructive pulmonary disease. Psychiatric patients who smoke are at increased risk for death from smoking-related diseases. Further, smoking can result in fires in clinical and residential settings. Fifty percent of smokers die prematurely (Peto 1994); in addition, more than 20% of all deaths in the United States are attributed to smoking (McGinnis and Foege 1993). Individuals successfully recovering from alcohol dependence are more likely to die from smoking-related diseases than from alcohol-related diseases (Hurt 1996).

Three sets of comprehensive guidelines—from the American Psychiatric Association (APA) (1996), the Agency for Health Care Policy and Research (AHCPR) (1996), and the U.S. Preventive Services Task Force (PSTF) (1996)—are now available to help clinicians increase their knowledge of nicotine addiction and, more important, to develop treatment skills in this area. The guidelines are complementary and provide three valuable perspectives on the assessment and treatment of tobacco addiction.

The PSTF and AHCPR guidelines describe the core approaches that could be used in any health care setting. They are designed for primary care clinicians who have little specialized training in behavioral therapies or psychotropic medications. The guidelines are also useful for psychiatrists doing consultation-liaison work in primary care settings.

The APA guidelines provide detailed recommendations for

blending pharmacological and behavioral therapies to treat smokers with more complicated cases, such as an individual with heavy nicotine dependence as well as psychiatric and substance abuse problems. Chronic smokers who are not able to stop smoking often require more intensive treatments (AHCPR 1996; APA 1996). The APA guidelines can be obtained by calling 1-800-368-5777; the AHCPR guidelines can be obtained by calling 1-800-358-9295. Another excellent resource is *Nicotine Addiction: Principles and Management* (Orleans and Slade 1993).

Barriers to implementing treatment for nicotine dependence in mental health settings include clinicians' fears of exacerbating the psychiatric disorder, lack of training in smoking cessation, belief that psychiatric patients are not interested and cannot quit, use of smoking as a behavioral reinforcer in treatment, and the nonpayment of smoking cessation treatment services and medications. Smoking cessation services and medications should be reimbursed by health insurance plans (Goldstein 1997).

Epidemiology of Nicotine Use

Currently, about 25% of the general population are smokers (U.S. Department of Health and Human Services 1996). The overall prevalence of smoking has declined since the Surgeon General's report in the 1960s, but this decline is unequal across sociodemographic groups. About 49% of those who "ever smoked" have quit. Nonetheless, as the prevalence of smoking declines in the general population, the percentage of "hard-core" smokers increases, a phenomenon that may slow the rate of decline in smoking (Goldstein et al. 1991; Pierce 1989). Higher rates of smoking are associated with female gender, white race, lower educational level, and lower socioeconomic levels (U.S. Department of Health and Human Services 1996).

Current estimates reveal an average of 3,000 new smokers— mostly adolescents—per day. More than 3 million adolescents smoke, including 28% of high-school seniors, and more than 1 million adolescent males use smokeless tobacco. By age 18, 90% of those who will ever try a cigarette have done so, and the average age at which individuals become daily smokers is 17.7 years.

Among the many risk factors for adolescent tobacco use are lower levels of school achievement, lower self-esteem than non-tobacco-using peers, poorer self-image, higher dropout rates, fewer skills to resist peer pressure to use tobacco, comorbid conduct and/or attention deficit disorders, and more involvement in other high-risk behaviors (Goldstein et al. 1991).

The National Health Interview Survey found that 70% of smokers interviewed reported that they wanted to quit smoking at some point in their lifetimes. Although about 33% of smokers try to quit each year, less than 10% are able to complete 1 year of total abstinence. Most quitters relapse within days. Among 1-year quitters, 33% have relapses. Motivation predicts outcome and relative treatment intensity.

Smoking is very common among psychiatric patients and/or substance abuse patients. Smoking rates among these patients are two to three times those among the general population. The rates of smoking are similar among patients with schizophrenia (69%–88%), affective disorders or mania (55%–70%), alcohol dependence (70%–90%), and other drug abuse (70%–95%) (Hughes 1986; Ziedonis et al. 1994).

Basic Pharmacology

Nicotine is readily absorbed from tobacco smoke in the lungs and from smokeless tobacco in the mouth and nose (U.S. Department of Health and Human Services 1988). On average, about 0.5–2.0 mg of nicotine is absorbed from each cigarette. Some smokers are more effective than others at extracting nicotine from cigarettes while smoking. Chewing tobacco can deliver up to 4.5 mg and a pinch of snuff about 3.5 mg of nicotine. The half-life of nicotine is about 90–120 minutes. Nicotine rapidly accumulates in the brain during smoking, producing peak brain concentrations within 1 minute. Both the speed and the extent of nicotine's effects on the brain lead to reinforcement and drug dependence. Not surprisingly, individuals develop a tolerance to nicotine use (Henningfield et al. 1985).

Nicotine is a psychostimulant with dose-dependent biphasic effects. In the brain, nicotine activates nicotinic acetylcholine receptors, increasing the neuronal firing rate and the smoker's feelings of alertness. Nicotine then produces desensitization to nicotinic acetylcholine receptors and reduces the firing rate, which results in a sense of relaxation. Through presynaptic mechanisms, nicotine increases the metabolism and release of dopamine in the brain reward pathway, resulting in feelings of pleasure and relaxation (Henningfield et al. 1985; U.S. Department of Health and Human Services 1988).

Nicotine has a wide variety of stimulant (with lower doses) and depressant (with higher doses) effects involving the central and peripheral nervous systems, cardiovascular and endocrine systems, and other systems (U.S. Department of Health and Human Services 1988). Effects on the peripheral nervous system include skeletal muscle relaxation through ganglionic blockade. Effects on the central nervous system include electrocortical activation and increases in brain serotonin, endogenous opioid peptides, pituitary hormones, catecholamines, and vasopressin, which result in enhancement of pleasure, task performance, and memory; reduction of anxiety, tension, and pain; and avoidance of weight gain (Pomerleau and Pomerleau 1984; U.S. Department of Health and Human Services 1988). Nicotine increases attention, memory, and learning in smokers, especially when the tasks are boring and long and the desire for stimulation is at its peak (Levin 1992).

Perhaps due to nicotine's effect on cholinergic pathways controlling cortical activation and arousal, it appears to improve general attention-processing capacity, that is, selective and sustained attention and the ability to disregard irrelevant stimuli, particularly under situations of stress or cognitive deficits. Nicotine has positive effects on mood regulation, affect, and stress. Some researchers are evaluating the role of maintenance nicotine replacement for psychiatric patients quitting smoking and for nonsmoking patients who might benefit from nicotine's effects (Goldstein et al. 1991; Jarvik 1991).

Tobacco contains many compounds in addition to nicotine. Unprocessed tobacco smoke includes more than 2,500 compounds, and when manufactured additives and other compounds are taken into account, there are about 4,000 compounds present

(U.S. Department of Health and Human Services 1988). These compounds include carbon monoxide, carbon dioxide, ammonia, acetaldehyde, formaldehyde, and cyanide, to name a few, as well as unidentified, nonnicotine components of cigarette smoke that inhibit monoamine oxidase A and B (Fowler 1996), which may potentiate the rewarding effects of nicotine. Some clinicians prefer the term *tobacco addiction* rather than *nicotine dependence* to reflect the belief that some of these other compounds are psychoactive and may be reinforcing.

Nicotine Dependence

The diagnosis of nicotine dependence, as outlined by DSM-IV (APA 1994), is similar to that of the other drugs of abuse. In most cases, the criterion of tolerance and withdrawal are easily established in the daily smoker. Many smokers will describe unsuccessful previous attempts to cut down on their use of cigarettes. Contrary to other substances of abuse, cigarettes can be obtained quickly and easily; however, the advent of nonsmoking areas may result in the dependent smoker's devoting a significant amount of time and effort to finding an area where smoking is permitted. Consistent with the general growth in society's intolerance of smoking, patients may formulate their plans around whether smoking is permitted. They may reduce or eliminate their involvement in an activity that had previously been important because it does not allow them to satisfy their compulsion to smoke. Last and most important, they might continue to use nicotine in the face of significant physical problems that are worsened by smoking or are a direct result of smoking. Most tobacco smokers easily meet criteria for nicotine dependence. In fact, there is no DSM-IV diagnosis of nicotine abuse.

Another measure of nicotine dependence is the Fagerstrom Test for Nicotine Dependence (FTND) (Table 1–1; Heatherton et al. 1991), a revision of the original Fagerstrom Tolerance Scale. With its proven reliability and validity, the FTND is a tool often used in treatment studies. A score of 5 or higher on the FTND is indicative of nicotine dependence and suggests the need for higher-intensity psychosocial treatment and higher-dose nicotine replacement.

Table 1–1. Items and scoring for Fagerstrom test for nicotine dependence

Questions	Answer	Points
1. How soon after you wake up do you smoke your first cigarette?	Within 5 minutes	3
	6–30 minutes	2
	31–60 minutes	1
	After 60 minutes	0
2. Do you find it difficult to refrain from smoking in places where it is forbidden, such as in church, at the library, in the cinema, etc.?	Yes	1
	No	0
3. Which cigarette would you hate most to give up?	The first one in the morning	1
	All others	0
4. How many cigarettes per day do you smoke?	10 or fewer	0
	11–20	1
	21–30	2
	31 or more	3
5. Do you smoke more frequently during the first hours of waking than during the rest of the day?	Yes	1
	No	0
6. Do you smoke if you are so ill that you are in bed most of the day?	Yes	1
	No	0

Source. Adapted from American Psychiatric Association: *Practice Guideline for the Treatment of Patients With Nicotine Dependence.* Washington, D.C., American Psychiatric Association, 1996.

From a neurobiological perspective, there is strong evidence that the rewarding effects of smoking and nicotine dependence are mediated through the dopamine reward pathway, the mesolimbic dopamine system (Balfour and Fagerstrom 1996). This subset of dopamine neurons projects from the ventral tegmental area in the midbrain to terminal fields in the nucleus accumbens. The mesolimbic dopamine pathways are thought to subserve the rewarding, reinforcing, and motivating aspects of nicotine use. The presence of nicotinic acetylcholine receptors, the site of action of nicotine, has been found on mesolimbic dopamine neurons (Clarke and Pert 1985). Experimental studies in rodents have demonstrated that nicotine administration augments dopamine release in the nucleus accumbens (Pontieri et al. 1996), an effect also seen with other substances of abuse, such as cocaine, morphine, and alcohol. Other dopamine pathways, including the nigrostriatal and mesocortical projections, may also play a role in nicotine dependence (Ziedonis and George 1997). As such, nonrewarding factors, such as modulation of mood states (i.e. dysphoria), stress reduction, alleviation of side effects of psychotropic medication, and cognitive enhancement, may contribute to nicotine dependence, especially in psychiatric patients (Levin 1992; Ziedonis and George 1997).

Nicotine Withdrawal

Clinically, nicotine withdrawal has been well characterized. Subjective symptoms include dysphoric or depressed mood, often with associated irritability, anxiety, decreased concentration, and restlessness. The objective symptoms may include decreased heart rate (approximate decrease of eight beats per minute), weight gain (mean gain of 2–3 kg) secondary to increased appetite, and insomnia. The DSM-IV criterion of withdrawal requires four or more of these symptoms that are sufficiently severe to cause distress in the patient's normal life and that are not attributable to some other physical or mental illness. Other common symptoms not noted by DSM-IV include the craving, urge, or desire for nicotine and a desire for sweets. Patients may show signs of withdrawal, such as increased coughing, and impaired performance on vigilance tasks. Diagnostic tests may show slowing on electroencephalogram, sleep electroencephalographic changes, decreased cortisol and catecholamine levels, and a general decline in metabolic rate (APA 1996).

There is a relatively small body of literature on the biology of the nicotine withdrawal state. Evidence from both animals and humans points to abnormalities in catecholaminergic neurotransmission, particularly in terms of reduced dopaminergic and adrenergic and/or norepinephrine function (Fung et al. 1996; Ward et al. 1991). There may also be a role for serotonergic, cholinergic, endogenous opiate and hypothalamic-pituitary-adrenal function (Benwell and Balfour 1979; Malin et al. 1994). This basic pharmacological and neurobiological evidence points to strategies for the rational design of pharmacological therapies to facilitate smoking cessation.

Assessment Issues

All patients should be asked about their current and past patterns of tobacco and nicotine use, including multiple sources of nicotine (tobacco products and over-the-counter nicotine replacements). Smokers should be assessed for nicotine dependence and withdrawal, as well as for their prior attempts to quit, their current motivation to quit, barriers to quitting, and their preferences in treatment. Consideration should be given to the use of objective lab tests such as carbon monoxide or cotinine. In assessing quitting history, the clinician should ask about patients' numbers of quit attempts ever and in the past year, their use of nicotine replacement or other medications, whether they have ever enrolled in a formal smoking cessation program such as that of the American Lung Association, and how long they were able to stay abstinent. A comprehensive assessment also includes assessing patients' demographic and comorbid medical and psychiatric problems (especially depression and alcohol dependence), the time of last cigarette and withdrawal symptoms, their perceived health risks, their reasons for quitting (which could be assessed with the 20-item Reason for Quitting Scale [Curry 1993]), their perceived difficulty of quitting, and their interest in treatment and their preference for a specific strategy for smoking cessation. This information is important to decisions regarding treatment matching (APA 1996).

Both the patient's level of motivation (desire and readiness to quit) and self-efficacy (perceived ability to quit) should be assessed. The patient's reasons for wanting to quit smoking should be clarified; both the positive and the negative reasons for smoking will be addressed in the formulation of an individualized plan. A nonjudgmental assessment of these reasons may also improve the patient's motivation and increase the chances for successful abstinence.

One tool used to assess the Prochaska and DiClemente (1992) stages of change (precontemplation, contemplation, preparation, action, and maintenance) is the Contemplation Ladder (Bierner and Abrams 1991). In the precontemplation stage, the smoker is not interested in quitting smoking. In the contemplation stage, he continues to smoke; although he admits that he has a problem, he is not ready to stop smoking for about 6–12 months. In the preparation stage, the smoker continues to smoke but would like to quit in the next month. She might have made a few random, unsuccessful efforts to stop using substances, but she does not have a quit plan to guide her. In the action stage, the smoker is motivated to stop using and is willing to participate in treatment in order to develop an organized plan to do so. In the maintenance phase, the individual has been able to abstain from smoking for more than 3 months.

A large number of smokers, approximately 40%, have no intention of quitting. However, evidence from one large study showed that the inquiry alone on the part of the physician improved abstinence rates by 5% (APA 1996). Another study reported that 40% of smokers are ambivalent about stopping. A more in-depth assessment of the ambivalent patient may actually be enlightening and may increase the patient's motivation toward abstinence in the future. Lastly, 20% of all smokers at any one time are reportedly motivated to quit. They should receive a full assessment in order to develop an effective treatment plan and to enhance their motivation to quit.

A discussion of the barriers to smoking cessation can be clarified in the formal motivational assessment. Issues around previous experiences of mood change and anxiety can be noted for future reference and assistance in individualizing treatment. The clinician should also consider the timing of the patient's attempt to quit smoking. Of course, there may never be a perfect time to quit, but to attempt abstinence at a time of increased stress or dysphoria may doom the treatment to failure.

Patients may present with a desire for a particular therapy. This desire may be related to several factors: previous treatment failures or near successes; knowledge of a new approach noted in the lay press or related by a peer; or a stronger motivation to pursue a specific therapeutic approach. Some patients do not want to take nicotine replacement (saying, for example, "that's what I am trying to stop using"). Naturally, the clinician should consider the patient's preferences, addressing treatment pros and cons to establish clinical expertise and build a more solid therapeutic alliance with the patient.

Treatment for Nicotine Dependence

General Issues in Starting Treatment

Psychiatrists and other mental health specialists should ask all patients about their use of tobacco. When necessary, they should advise patients to stop and should personally assist them in quitting. The four A's of the National Cancer Institute remind us to Ask everyone about smoking, Advise smokers to quit, Assist those interested in quitting, and Arrange follow-up. Throughout this process, the importance of the therapeutic alliance should be remembered. Clinicians must remember that smoking is a chronic, relapsing addiction and can be difficult to extinguish. Patients should be approached with empathy and support with a view toward helping them through multiple attempts before they finally stop smoking (Prochaska and Goldstein 1991).

The clinician can start with a simple treatment approach and work to set a quit date. He or she should consider available resources, such as behavioral therapists, American Lung Association groups, and smoking cessation clinics. Brief advice should be provided and a motivational interviewing style used (to be described). The AHCPR/National Cancer Institute/APA guidelines focus on increasing the patient's motivation to make a quit attempt. The clinician should pick a time to stop (a quit date) when the patient is not in a crisis. He or she should then closely monitor the patient for worsening of psychiatric symptoms and changes in medication levels. Strategies to get reimbursed include requesting reimbursement for monitoring and treating "shortness of breath" (ICD-9 code system) or recurrent depression or anxiety when using smoking cessation methods.

For those smokers who have failed a first-line therapy, important factors to assess include the presence of psychiatric or substance abuse comorbidity, adequacy of first therapy, and any problems or side effects. In addition, reasons for the relapse should be established (e.g., a family member smokes, work environment, mood/irritability during withdrawal, and other triggers). Did the patient achieve any abstinence? If so, for how long?

Specific recommended psychosocial and pharmacological treatments are outlined in Table 1–2. First-line treatments include

Table 1–2. Recommended treatments for nicotine dependence

Psychosocial therapies
Multicomponent therapies
Behavioral therapies/relapse prevention
Motivational enhancement therapy
Brief advice
Self-help materials
Disease management programs (pharmaceutical industry programs)

Pharmacological therapies
Nicotine gum
Nicotine patch
Combination nicotine gum and patch
Bupropion (Zyban)
Nicotine nasal spray

brief advice, behavior therapy, nicotine patch or gum, and bupropion. Second-line treatments include more intensive behavioral therapies, nicotine patch plus gum, higher nicotine patch dosing, nicotine nasal spray, or nicotine inhaler. The psychosocial treatments include multicomponent therapies that blend skills training and relapse prevention, stimulus control, rapid smoking, self-help materials, and disease management programs (pharmaceutical industry programs). These approaches are well described in the APA Nicotine Treatment Guidelines (1996).

It is important to educate patients about withdrawal symptoms. Not only will patients learn to expect and recognize these symptoms as a natural part of withdrawal, but they will also view the symptoms as time-limited. Timing of quitting is often an important point for the patient. Though the adage "there is no time like the present" may be important in not allowing continued procrastination on the patient's part, there is reason to carefully plan out the quit date and help the patient to be well prepared for that time. One can then make sure that adequate care is taken to educate the patient, explore potential difficulties in quitting, and build the patient's motivation and sense of self-efficacy.

If the patient has ongoing psychiatric problems, the physician must weigh the level of present symptomatology, and the prospect of perhaps waiting until the patient is more stable, against the patient's current motivational level to quit. One should evaluate whether the patient's medications are known to be affected by nicotine usage (Table 1–3). The nonnicotine components of tobacco (smoke) often increase the metabolism of medications metabolized through the 1A2 isoenzyme of the P450 system. Thus, the blood level of some psychotropic medications rises with abstinence and falls with increased tobacco use. A dosage adjustment may be required in these instances (Balfour and Fagerstrom 1996).

One question that patients often ask physicians is whether to gradually reduce the number of cigarettes or to quit abruptly. There is no clear evidence that one technique is more effective than the other (Cinciripini et al. 1995; Law and Tang 1995). Patient preference is an important factor in the decision.

Weight gain, often encountered with smoking cessation, is a common concern of people anticipating abstinence. There is nor-

Table 1–3. Effect of abstinence from smoking on blood levels of medication

Effect of abstinence on blood levels	Medication
Increases	Clozapine
	Desipramine
	Desmethyldiazepam
	Doxepin
	Fluphenazine
	Haloperidol
	Imipramine
	Olanzapine
	Oxazepam
	Propranolol
Does not increase	Amitriptyline
	Bupropion
	Chlordiazepoxide
	Ethanol
	Lorazepam
	Midazolam
	Triazolam
Unclear	Alprazolam
	Chlorpromazine
	Diazepam

mally no more than a 2- to 3-kg weight gain, and this usually takes place in the first 3 months. Those most at risk for weight gain are women already trying to lose weight. Some individuals may find nicotine gum helpful to temporarily diminish this weight gain. Suggestions of increased activity and low-fat, nutritious diets can be helpful. The clinician may reiterate that the weight gain is usually not severe and certainly not as harmful to one's overall health as smoking. This may help to maintain the patient's motivation to quit. Patients should be advised not to diet because this may increase their chance of a smoking relapse.

Specific Psychosocial Treatments

Although there is great interest in the new pharmacotherapy options, treatment of smokers with comorbidity and severe nicotine dependence usually requires psychosocial treatments. The APA guidelines provide an excellent overview of the specific psychosocial treatments for smoking cessation that are listed in Table 1–2. Many of the psychosocial treatment approaches are similar to those for other chemical dependencies, but there are unique differences. Few abusers of nonnicotine drugs progress in their recovery without relatively long-term involvement in 12-step programs or some type of substance abuse treatment program, most of which are abstinence oriented and many of which are non-pharmacologically oriented. In contrast, smokers are often given only brief advice and nicotine replacement medications. Behavior therapy is very effective but is underutilized. In contrast to other addictions, there are numerous medical agencies (American Lung Association, American Heart Association, National Cancer Institute, etc.) that are invested in helping people stop smoking as a prevention effort to reduce the associated medical comorbidities. Smoking cessation psychosocial treatments are similar in using motivational interviewing and/or motivational enhancement therapy approaches and relapse prevention (identifying cues or triggers to use and developing coping techniques to manage those cues and triggers), but the 12-step programs are not core treatment modalities for nicotine dependence, as they are for other addictions.

Treatment matching. Other promising psychotherapy approaches include matching treatment to motivational level, comorbid psychiatric problem, and severity of dependence. Given the role of brief advice as the minimum acceptable level of psychosocial intervention, availability of over-the-counter products, and the competition among pharmaceutical companies for nicotine replacement options, excellent disease management programs (i.e., the American Lung Association's Freedom From Smoking [FFS] Programs) have been developed for consumers. These help busy primary care practitioners who have limited time, training, and resources to integrate behavioral therapies into the treatment plan. Treatment matching also considers the issue of low dose versus intensive treatment, increasing the intensity of psychosocial treatments with repeated smoking cessation efforts, and addressing comorbid psychiatric problems. Other approaches include skills training, and behavioral strategies to avoid triggers, decrease withdrawal symptoms, and develop new coping strategies.

Motivational interventions. Most smokers (about 80%) are not currently motivated to quit and need motivational interventions. The motivational intervention actually begins with the assessment of the patient's own reasons for seeing a physician, which can be materially useful in building the motivation to quit. One needs to provide information on elements of the patient's biopsychosocial health that may be affected by continuing to smoke. One must also offer clarity, empathy, and empowerment to the patient, thus fostering the need for change. It is equally important, however, that one discuss the perceived positive role that the use of tobacco has had in the patient's life. If this area is not addressed, the patient will be asked to give up a valuable part of his or her life with no discussion of how to replace it.

Such a discussion may require only a few minutes or may require multiple sessions carried out in small increments over a period of months or years while treating the patient for other problems. By making it a part of the treatment plan, one can return to the subject repeatedly and thus continue to build awareness over time. Needless to say, patient self-efficacy is an important treatment issue. Most patients will have already attempted to quit. Thus, they will have some experience with failure. Patients should be advised that most successful quitters have to make multiple (more than five) attempts before they achieve abstinence; thus, it is important to combat patient discouragement. Relapse prevention behavior therapy focuses on developing self-efficacy to manage specific triggers to smoking.

Pharmacological Approaches to Smoking Cessation

As in all areas of psychiatry, combining pharmacotherapies and psychotherapies is important and leads to improved outcomes. Outcomes also improve with more intensive psychosocial interventions. The pharmacological approaches to smoking cessation that have been approved by the U.S. Food and Drug Administration (FDA) include nicotine replacement therapies (i.e., patch, gum, spray, and inhaler) and bupropion. These products aim to reduce withdrawal symptoms and the desire for nicotine. Non-FDA-approved options (e.g., clonidine, buspirone) target reducing the effects of nicotine withdrawal, blocking the effects of nicotine (e.g., mecamylamine), or causing an aversive reaction (e.g., silver acetate).

In this section, we discuss current and possible pharmacotherapies for smoking cessation with these strategies in mind. This topic has been reviewed elsewhere (Balfour and Fagerstrom 1996). Patient preference is an important factor in considering medication options. Some patients prefer a particular route of administration (pill, patch, gum, spray, or inhaler), whereas others may not want to receive nicotine replacement at all. Brief advice should include reviewing all FDA-approved options and instilling hope that multiple options are possible if the first effort does not succeed.

Nicotine replacement therapy.   Nicotine replacement strategies are based on the principle that nicotine is the dependence-producing constituent of cigarette smoking and that smoking cessation and abstinence can be achieved by replacing nicotine without the harmful impurities in cigarette smoke. There are slow-acting (nicotine patch), intermediate-acting (nicotine gum and inhaler), and fast-acting (spray) delivery strategies. However, all of these methods are significantly less efficient in nicotine delivery than is smoking cigarettes. Nicotine patch and gum are now available over the counter and will probably be the first-line medication choices of many smokers attempting to quit on their own. Given the safety profile and efficacy of nicotine replacement, all patients should be offered nicotine replacement as a viable treatment option. Of note is that the abuse liability of nicotine replacement appears to be minimal (APA 1996; Pickworth 1994; Schuh 1997).

The nicotine transdermal patch produces a ready absorption of nicotine through the skin; however, it does not allow for self-titrated dosing for craving and nicotine withdrawal symptoms. The patch is convenient to use and produces less fluctuation in plasma nicotine levels. The available brands of nicotine patch begin at 15, 21, and 22 mg, and lower doses of 7 and 14 mg are used to taper the patch after smoking cessation. The available brands include Nicotrol (15 mg/day), Nicoderm (21 mg/day), Habitrol (21 mg/day), and ProStep (22 mg/day). All patches deliver approximately 0.9 mg of nicotine per hour. Steady-state nicotine levels are 13–25 ng/ml, and the highest levels are seen soon after patch application. This amount is about half that delivered by smoking a cigarette. There have been more than 20 placebo-controlled trials of the nicotine patch in smoking cessation (reviewed by Balfour and Fagerstrom 1996), which generally demonstrate excellent short-term (6-week) abstinence rates (40% versus 20%) but more modest long-term (1-year) rates (19% versus 10%). Common side effects of the patch include local skin reactions at the site of application, myalgias (rare), and sleep disturbances with the 24-hour patch. The nicotine patch has been recommended to be used for a total of 6–12 weeks (APA 1996).

Nicotine polacrilex gum was the first available nicotine replacement therapy for smoking cessation. It is available in doses of 2 mg and 4 mg; recommended dosing is in the range of 9–16 pieces per day, and heavy smokers (more than 25 cigarettes per day) often require the 4-mg dose. It seems to be most effective when used frequently (i.e., hourly). Peak blood nicotine levels achieved are low (approximately 10–15 ng/ml) compared with those in dependent smokers (15–100 ng/ml). Many smokers state that nicotine gum may help reduce nicotine craving, but generally it does not significantly curtail nicotine withdrawal symptoms (Balfour and Fagerstrom 1996). In controlled studies, the nicotine patch may result in quit rates that are double those produced by placebo gum (Fagerstrom 1994; Hughes 1993). Side effects of the gum include local irritation in the mouth, throat, and stomach; nausea; indigestion; and jaw muscle soreness.

Nicotine nasal spray is the most recent nicotine replacement modality to be approved by the FDA and is a prescription drug. Smokers are advised to use this spray as needed, as for gum. A single dose of the spray delivers 0.5 mg to each nostril, and it can be used one to three times per hour. It has been suggested that the effective daily dose in nicotine-dependent smokers is 15–20 sprays (8–10 mg) per day (Balfour and Fagerstrom 1996). Onset of action of the spray is the most rapid of all nicotine replacements; nicotine levels in plasma reach 10–20 ng/ml. Because the drug is absorbed through the nasal mucosa into the arterial circulation, it is estimated to reach the brain within 10 seconds (Balfour and Fagerstrom 1996). The three placebo-controlled studies to date (Schneider 1995) support the efficacy of the spray in long-term treatment of smoking cessation: Quit rates with the nicotine spray were double those with placebo spray. Side effects of the spray include local airway irritation (i.e., coughing, rhinorrhea, lacrimation, nasal irritation), but tolerance to these local effects appears to develop. Systemic effects include nausea, headache, dizziness, tachycardia, and sweating (Balfour and Fagerstrom 1996). It has been shown that addition of the nicotine spray does not increase myocardial oxygen demand in cigarette smokers (Keeley et al. 1996), making it safe in smokers with cardiovascular disease. The nicotine spray may have rewarding effects in smokers (Perkins 1997). However, the abuse liability appears to be minimal (Schuh 1997).

Nicotine vapor inhaler is delivered through a mouthpiece with a plug saturated with nicotine and menthol to mask the aversive taste of nicotine and reduce local irritation. It is used much like an inhaler for bronchial asthma and may mimic the upper airway stimulation derived by habitual smokers; however, absorption is mostly buccal and not respiratory (APA 1996); therefore it is actually not a true inhaler. The amount of nicotine delivered is effort dependent and substantially less (0.013 mg per inhalation) than that delivered by the nicotine spray (Schuh 1997); users must puff quite vigorously to administer satisfying nicotine doses. Plasma nicotine levels are about 8–10 ng/ml. Excluding the levels achieved with the nicotine patch, these levels are lower than those produced by other nicotine replacements. Controlled trials (Schneider 1996b) indicate 1-year abstinence rates of 17% for the nicotine inhaler and 8% for placebo. Side effects include cough, throat irritation, nausea, headache, and dyspepsia. Abuse liability appears to be minimal (Schuh 1997).

Bupropion. The first FDA-approved nonnicotine replacement therapy, bupropion (Zyban; Nides 1997) is the only such medication that is FDA approved for treating nicotine dependence. This heterocyclic, atypical antidepressant modestly blocks the reuptake of both dopamine and norepinephrine. The efficacy of bupropion as an aid to smoking cessation was demonstrated in three double-blind, placebo-controlled trials in nondepressed chronic cigarette smokers (Hurt 1997). Smoking cessation rates appear to improve further when the drug is combined with the nicotine patch (Nides 1997).

Early trials demonstrated that bupropion (300 mg/day) could enhance smoking cessation rates in depressed and nondepressed smokers. In a recent multicenter study of 615 smokers, Hurt (1997) reported that sustained-release bupropion significantly enhanced smoking cessation rates after 7 weeks of treatment. The study also demonstrated that the effects of bupropion were dose dependent: abstinence rates at 6 weeks were 19.0%, 28.8%, 38.6%, and 44.2% for groups receiving placebo, 100 mg/day, 150 mg/day, and 300 mg/day, respectively. Further, weight gain from smoking cessation was inversely related to bupropion dose, but this agent did not significantly alter nicotine withdrawal symptoms.

In all studies, adverse events had a low incidence and included dry mouth, insomnia, nausea, and skin rash. In the treatment of depression, the occurrence of seizures was found to be dose dependent, similar to that associated with other antidepressants, and was not considered to be of significant risk (0.1%–0.4% at

300–450 mg/day) unless the daily dose of bupropion exceeded 450 mg/day. There have been no reports of seizure in any smoking cessation studies to date. Nonetheless, this agent should not be used in patients with a history of seizure disorder. The effects of bupropion in smoking cessation appear to be unrelated to its antidepressant properties (Hurt 1997).

Non-FDA-approved medication strategies.   The experience with nonapproved, nonnicotine replacement strategies is limited, but an increasing number of controlled studies have evaluated such agents. These drugs are thought to target mechanisms underlying the initiation and maintenance of both nicotine dependence and withdrawal, particularly with respect to monoaminergic function. The use of psychotropic agents in smoking cessation is supported by the high rates of comorbid nicotine dependence in patients with psychiatric disorders (Glassman 1993; Hughes 1986), particularly affective disorders (Covey et al. 1997) and schizophrenia (George et al. 1995; McEvoy et al. 1995; Ziedonis and George 1997).

Clonidine, an antihypertensive and sympatholytic agent, is a presynaptic α2-receptor agonist that has been used extensively in the management of opiate and alcohol withdrawal. Clonidine is available in both oral (0.1 mg) and transdermal patch (0.1- to 0.3-mg) forms. This agent has been shown to dose-dependently reduce nicotine withdrawal and craving (Gourlay 1994), but benefits may be confined to female smokers (Glassman et al. 1988) and may be effective only when combined with behavior modification (Hilleman 1994). Sedation, orthostatic hypotension, sexual dysfunction, and fatigue are common but serious side effects and can be minimized with use of the transdermal patch preparation.

Buspirone is a nonsedating, nonbenzodiazepine, anxiolytic agent indicated for the treatment of generalized anxiety. There is some limited evidence (Cinciripini 1995; Schneider 1996a) that it can reduce nicotine craving and has limited efficacy in promoting smoking cessation, although one report suggests that it may be as effective as the patch when combined with behavior modification (Hilleman 1994). High doses (30–60 mg/day) may be needed, and patients with high levels of generalized anxiety (Cinciripini 1995) may preferentially benefit during smoking cessation attempts.

Other than the FDA-approved bupropion, the most promising antidepressants for smoking cessation appear to be nortriptyline and doxepin (Humfleet et al. 1996). The serotonin-selective reuptake inhibitors do not appear to have similar efficacy, even though serotonin may play a role in dysphoria (Dalack 1995) and the weight gain associated with nicotine withdrawal. However, one study of fluoxetine in depressed alcoholic smokers found that this serotonin-selective reuptake inhibitor reduced smoking and alcohol consumption.

Moclobemide is a reversible inhibitor of monoamine oxidase A that has been approved for the treatment of major depression in Canada and Europe. Because it increases the synaptic availability of monoamines (dopamine, norepinephrine, and 5-hydroxytryptamine [serotonin]), it may have benefit in smoking cessation. Further, because a component in cigarette smoke other than nicotine inhibits both monoamine oxidase A and B activity (Fowler 1996), such agents may have a further effect on smoking cessation. Moclobemide has been shown to be effective in smoking cessation in highly dependent smokers at 6 and 12 months after quit date (Berlin 1995), and this finding deserves further evaluation.

Atypical antipsychotic agents may help patients with schizophrenia to reduce their smoking and improve their chances at smoking cessation by better treating negative symptoms, cognitive deficits, and medication side effects. Two preliminary studies (George et al. 1995; McEvoy et al. 1995) suggest that clozapine reduces nicotine craving and smoking consumption, and this may relate to level of nicotine dependence (George et al. 1995) and clozapine plasma levels (McEvoy et al. 1995).

Silver acetate is a deterrent therapy (like disulfiram [Antabuse] for alcohol dependence) that interacts with cigarette smoke to produce an unpleasant metallic taste. It is available over the counter in both lozenge and gum forms; a mouth spray has also been studied. There is some evidence of efficacy in smoking cessation, particularly in smokers with a limited history of nicotine dependence. The dose is 6 mg up to six times daily. Side effects include silver toxicity and skin discoloration.

Combining medications. Compliance with taking one medication can be an issue, but the potential advantages of combining medications may be an important advance for chronic smokers who have been unsuccessful with the nicotine patch or gum alone. Increasing the overall dose of nicotine replacement may help smokers with heavy dependence. From clinical experience, some heavy smokers or smokers who demonstrate intense nicotine withdrawal symptoms appear to benefit from using nicotine patch doses in the range of 28–42 mg.

Another strategy is to combine the patch with other nicotine replacement medications. The rationale behind combined nicotine replacement approaches is to exploit both the reward effects of fast onset, like nicotine gum (thus mimicking the positive reinforcing effects of nicotine derived from smoking), and to alternate withdrawal symptoms through steady levels of nicotine produced by slow-acting forms such as the nicotine patch. The best of these combinations studied is that of nicotine gum and patch. Two studies (Kornitzer 1995; Puska 1995) have found a modest (1.5-fold; 21% versus 14%) increase in efficacy for 1-year abstinence rates for the gum-patch combination over gum alone. Given the enhanced bioavailability and rapid onset of action of the nicotine spray, its combination with the nicotine patch may be even more effective.

Although few studies have combined nicotine replacement with nonnicotine replacement strategies, this would seem like a reasonable therapeutic strategy because multiple neurobiological mechanisms of action would, in theory, be utilized. One trial compared sustained-release bupropion with a placebo patch, nicotine patch (Habitrol System, Parke-Davis) with placebo pills, sustained-release bupropion with nicotine patch, and placebo patch with placebo pills in nondepressed smokers. Patients treated with the combination of sustained-release bupropion and the nicotine patch achieved higher abstinence rates than did patients in each of the individual treatments alone (58%), although this result only approached significance ($P = .06$; Nides 1997).

Another study examined the combination of nicotine patch and mecamylamine (Rose et al. 1994) and found significantly increased effectiveness of the nicotine patch combined with mecamylamine over the nicotine patch alone at 7 weeks, 6 months, and 12 months. The authors suggested that the mechanism of action of this combination includes blockade of nicotine's reinforcing effects by mecamylamine and withdrawal relief by the nicotine patch treatment. Mecamylamine is a nonselective antagonist of high-affinity nicotinic acetylcholine receptors. The drug has been marketed as an antihypertensive (Inversine). In animal models, mecamylamine can precipitate nicotine withdrawal symptoms in dependent animals (Malin et al. 1994). When given to smokers, however, it does not precipitate nicotine withdrawal (Eissenberg et al. 1996), and thus may be acceptable during smoking cessation.

Other Somatic Treatments

Some individuals believe that acupuncture, hypnosis, and hypnotherapy have been very helpful in their smoking cessation efforts. However, controlled trials have not consistently shown the efficacy of these methods, and the APA guidelines determined that these treatments lacked sufficient evidence to be recommended (APA 1996).

Comorbidity of Nicotine Dependence With Psychiatric Illness

Why do so many psychiatric patients smoke? Potential biological factors include nicotine dependence (rewarding properties are greater in psychiatric patients), nicotine withdrawal (withdrawal is more severe and/or worsens symptoms in psychiatric patients), reduction of side effects of psychiatric medications (especially sedation and perhaps extrapyramidal symptoms), the stress-reducing effects of nicotine (especially in stress-responsive exacerbation of affective disorders and schizophrenia), and cognitive enhancement by nicotine (especially in prefrontal cortical dysfunction of schizophrenia). Potential psychosocial factors include self-medication to increase attention, alertness, and concentration or to reduce anxiety, depression, and boredom.

The mental health system has been a smoking-enriched environment in which patients and staff model and support smoking habits. Smoking is both a behavioral filler and a social connector for many psychiatric patients and may satisfy oral gratification needs and address body weight concerns. Psychiatric patients also tend to suffer from a lack of social activity, lower socioeconomic status, and unemployment (APA 1996).

Substance Abuse and Nicotine Use

Smoking rates among substance abusers are high, in the range of 75%–92% (Clemmey 1997). Heavy smoking is especially associated with alcohol and other drug abuse disorders. Substance abuse is also associated with difficulty in quitting smoking (Goldstein et al. 1991). Alcohol use is reported to be a significant precipitant of smoking relapse in the general population (Shiffman 1982), and continued smoking is negatively associated with long-term alcohol abstinence rates. Of interest is that about 50% of alcoholic persons express a strong desire to attend a smoking treatment program and many have made multiple attempts to quit.

Why is there a lack of interest in smoking cessation among addiction treatment programs? Perhaps staff in their own recovery have not addressed their own nicotine dependence and are less likely to address this in their patients. The recovery model emphasizes a developmental approach to recovery, and the early phases include abstinence from all substances except nicotine. Later stages of recovery do not include nicotine cessation and focus on addressing lifestyle changes, finding and developing healthy relationships, becoming more spiritually focused, and striving for overall self-improvement. Although conventional wisdom has argued against addressing tobacco dependence in the context of treating other addictions, this view is being challenged (Hughes 1993). A growing number of substance abuse programs have begun to offer some form of smoking cessation treatment (Clemmey 1997; Hoffman and Slade 1993).

Depression and Nicotine Use

Major depression and depressive symptoms are strongly associated with smoking and with severity of nicotine dependence. This association has important clinical implications for smoking cessation in primary care and psychiatric settings. The etiology of this association is most likely secondary to multiple biopsychosocial factors. Twin studies appear to demonstrate that smoking does not cause depression and depression does not cause smoking, but that shared genetic factors seem to predispose individuals to both smoking and depression (Kendler 1993).

In the general population, smokers are twice as likely as nonsmokers to have had a major depressive episode in their lifetimes (Glassman et al. 1988). The association with smoking is even stronger with recurrent major depression than with a single episode (Glassman 1993). There may be an increased risk of suicide in smokers versus nonsmokers. The risk for major depression increases with the severity of nicotine dependence (odds ratio = 1.9 with mild dependence versus 4.7 with moderate dependence; Breslau et al. 1991) and average number of cigarettes consumed (Kendler 1993).

About 25%–40% of smokers who enter smoking cessation programs have a history of major depression, and many have current dysthymic symptoms (Glassman 1993; Hall et al. 1993). Smokers with a history of depression are twice as likely as those without such a history to be unsuccessful at smoking cessation (14% versus 28%; Glassman et al. 1990). The poorer prognosis may be due to the fact that depressed smokers have more severe nicotine withdrawal symptoms (especially depressive symptoms) and are at risk for a relapse of depressive episode (Glassman 1997; Hall et al. 1993). About 25% of individuals with a history of major depression can have a severe depressive relapse during smoking cessation (Glassman 1997). In addition to having a history of major depression, experiencing severe negative mood and depressive symptoms during early nicotine withdrawal is strongly associated with smoking relapse (Covey et al. 1997; Hall et al. 1993).

Treatment Implications for Comorbidity of Substance Abuse and/or Depression With Nicotine Dependence

When assisting an individual in smoking cessation, the clinician should first screen for alcohol and drug abuse, depression, and anxiety disorders. Second, he or she should monitor drug abuse

---

and depressive symptoms during withdrawal and should be wary of a smoking relapse in vulnerable individuals. Third, the level of nicotine dependence should be assessed and the need for more intensive psychosocial and pharmacological treatment considered. Fourth, for individuals with a history of depression who are not currently taking an antidepressant, the use of an antidepressant during the smoking cessation period should be considered. Bupropion, nortriptyline, and doxepin might be first-line choices (Glassman 1997; Humfleet et al. 1996; Hurt 1997). Disulfiram and naltrexone might be considered for alcoholic patients. Fifth, more intensive psychosocial treatments that address relapse to smoking, alcohol/drug abuse, and depression should be considered. Although data from controlled trials are limited, combining cognitive-behavioral therapy for depression with an antidepressant improves smoking cessation outcomes in patients with a history of depression or depressive symptoms (Hall et al. 1994; Humfleet et al. 1996). Supportive counseling (such as Alcoholics Anonymous) may also be helpful (Zelman et al. 1992). Mood management may help smokers develop skills to identify and manage situations that lead to anger, anxiety, and depression. A central premise of this approach is that thoughts, activities, and mood interact to influence smoking behavior. Helpful techniques include relaxation training, thought-stopping, increasing pleasant activities, rational emotive techniques, and improving social support and social contacts.

Schizophrenia and Nicotine Use

Individuals with schizophrenia have high rates of smoking, in the range of 70%–90% (Glassman 1993; Hughes 1986; Ziedonis and George 1997; Ziedonis et al. 1994). Heavy nicotine use is associated with increased positive symptoms (Ziedonis et al. 1994) and increased (Goff et al. 1992) or decreased (Ziedonis et al. 1994) negative symptoms, reduced neuroleptic side effects, and increased nonnicotine substance abuse (Goff et al. 1992; Ziedonis et al. 1994). A recent study demonstrated that schizophrenic smokers are effective and efficient smokers who have higher urinary cotinine levels than do nonschizophrenic smokers (Olincy et al. 1997). Of interest is the finding that schizophrenic individuals have electrophysiological deficits in auditory gating related to the P50 response, which is known to be mediated by α7 nicotinic receptors in the hippocampus (Adler et al. 1993; Leonard 1996). There is evidence that nicotine administration via smoking can transiently normalize defective P50 potentials in schizophrenic patients and their nonschizophrenic relatives, and that a polymorphism in the α7 nicotinic receptor gene on chromosome 15 may be present in schizophrenic patients and their family members who have defective P50 auditory responses (Freedman 1997). These results suggest that defective P50 auditory-evoked responses may be an inheritable trait in schizophrenic patients and their nonschizophrenic relatives, that these deficits may be normalized by nicotine, and that this defect may contribute to increased smoking (to compensate for deficient hippocampal auditory processing) in schizophrenic patients. More study on the nature of this defect is required and may contribute to a better understanding of nicotine dependence in nonschizophrenic smokers and of the low-affinity α7 nicotinic receptor in normal brain function and neuropsychiatric disease.

The findings related to the α7 nicotinic receptor suggest that multiple forms of the nicotinic receptor (including the mecamylamine-sensitive, high-affinity nicotinic receptors containing the β subunit) may mediate nicotine's biobehavioral actions during both nicotine dependence and withdrawal and may have relevance to the pathophysiology of neuropsychiatric diseases such as schizophrenia. Given the potential benefits of nicotine in this population, some have suggested the use of maintenance nicotine replacement (i.e., long-acting nicotinic receptor agonists) as part of treatment for schizophrenia and for other smokers with heavy nicotine dependence (Warner et al. 1997). Although few studies on treatment for smoking cessation have been reported, given the severity of nicotine dependence and other psychosocial factors, early attempts at smoking cessation should include intensive psychosocial and pharmacological support (APA 1996).

Smoking Cessation in a Mental Health Center

The clinical experience of a smoking cessation program within a mental health center (Ziedonis and George 1997) has been reported for smokers with depression and schizophrenia. Patients were accepted into the program if their mental status was stable and there were no immediate plans to change their psychiatric medication or psychosocial treatment. All patients expressed interest in the program, but many who initially entered the program were relatively unmotivated to quit using immediately (50% were in the contemplation stage [Prochaska and DiClemente 1992]). During the initial weeks to months of the program, staff used motivational enhancement therapy to focus on the patients' own motivators and barriers to quitting smoking (decisional balance). Patients interested in quitting were recommended for nicotine patch and/or nicotine gum plus participation in a group behavior therapy program. Nicotine replacement was supplied free of charge. Bupropion was an option for patients who failed nicotine replacement or desired non-nicotine-based pharmacotherapy.

Patients were seen at multiple points after their quit date (2 days after and twice weekly after that) to monitor nicotine withdrawal, psychiatric symptoms, medication side effects, and blood levels. Successful outcomes (50% completed the program, 40% reduced smoking by one-half, and 13% had carbon monoxide–verified abstinence at 6 months) were associated with increased motivational levels, continued use of antidepressant or antipsychotic medication, receiving 4 weeks of motivational enhancement therapy prior to the quit date, starting nicotine replacement therapy on the quit date, and participating in 10 weeks of group treatment (modified American Lung Association and psychoeducation; relapse prevention, cognitive-behavioral therapy, and/or mood management; and support) (Ziedonis and George 1997). Some patients made several attempts to quit before achieving stable abstinence. Of note is that careful monitoring of side effects and blood levels of psychiatric medications identified increased sedation as a side effect that interfered with outcomes.

Treatment of Smokers on Smoke-Free Wards

The APA guidelines (1996) summarize the literature on managing smokers on a smoke-free unit. The smoking status of all patients should be documented, and smokers should have nicotine dependence on their problem list. Issues involved in managing nicotine dependence include educating patients about the rationale for smoke-free units, monitoring nicotine withdrawal symptoms, the potential impact of reduced smoking on medication blood levels, and the use of nicotine replacement to diagnose nicotine withdrawal and manage withdrawal symptoms. Of note is that, although the smoke in cigarettes affects medication blood levels, nicotine replacement does not. Policies for off-unit breaks and privileges should be similar for smokers and nonsmokers and should be based on psychiatric symptoms and risks for elopement. Patients should be educated about the public health need for smoke-free units, and smokers should be advised of the acute goal of managing nicotine withdrawal symptoms and asked to consider a long-term goal of quitting smoking.

Summary

Nicotine dependence through the use of tobacco products remains a serious public health problem, but recent clinical and preclinical research advances, coupled with timely policy changes, suggest novel and effective means for the treatment of smoking cessation at biological, psychological, and societal levels. Multiple nicotine replacement therapies, nonnicotine pharmacotherapies, and psychotherapeutic interventions, used most effectively in combination, offer hope to patients, particularly those with psychiatric illness, who find it hardest to stop smoking.

References

Adler LE, Hoffer LD, Wiser A, et al: Normalization of auditory physiology by cigarette smoking in schizophrenic patients. Am J Psychiatry 150:1856–1861, 1993
Agency for Health Care Policy and Research: Smoking cessation clinical practice guidelines. JAMA 275:1270–1280, 1996
American Psychiatric Association: Diagnostic and Statistical Manual of Mental Disorders, 4th Edition. Washington, DC, American Psychiatric Association, 1994

American Psychiatric Association: Practice Guideline for the Treatment of Patients With Nicotine Dependence. Washington, DC, American Psychiatric Association, 1996

Balfour DJK, Fagerstrom KO: Pharmacology of nicotine and its therapeutic use in smoking cessation and neurodegenerative disorders. Pharmacol Ther 72:51–81, 1996

Benwell MEM, Balfour DJK: Effects of nicotine administration and its withdrawal on plasma corticosterone and brain 5-hydroxyindoles. Psychopharmacology 63:7–11, 1979

Berlin I: A reversible monoamine oxidase A inhibitor (moclobemide) facilitates smoking cessation and abstinence in heavy, dependent smokers. Clin Pharmacol Ther 58:444–452, 1995

Bierner L, Abrams D: The contemplation ladder: validation of a measure of readiness to consider smoking cessation. Health Psychol 10:360–365, 1991

Breslau N, Kilbey M, Andreski P: Nicotine dependence, depression, and anxiety in young adults. Arch Gen Psychiatry 48:1069–1074, 1991

Cinciripini PM: A placebo-controlled evaluation of the effects of buspirone on smoking cessation: differences between high- and low-anxiety smokers. J Clin Psychopharmacol 15:182–191, 1995

Cinciripini PM, Lapitsky L, Seay S, et al: The effects of smoking schedules on cessation outcome: can we improve on common methods of gradual and abrupt nicotine withdrawal? J Consult Clin Psychol 63:388–399, 1995

Clarke PBS, Pert A: Autoradiographic evidence of nicotine receptors on nigrostriatal and mesolimbic dopamine neurons. Brain Res 348:355–358, 1985

Clemmey P: Smoking habits and attitudes in a methadone maintenance treatment population. Drug Alcohol Depend 44:123–132, 1997

Covey LS, Glassman AH, Stetner F: Major depression following smoking cessation. Am J Psychiatry 154:263–265, 1997

Curry SJ: Self-help interventions for smoking cessation. J Consult Clin Psychol 61:790–803, 1993

Dalack GW: Mood, major depression, and fluoxetine response in cigarette smokers. Am J Psychiatry 152:398–403, 1995

Eissenberg T, Griffiths RR, Stitzer ML: Mecamylamine does not precipitate withdrawal in cigarette smokers. Psychopharmacology 127:328–336, 1996

Fagerstrom KO: Review of nicotine gum and tailoring treatment to different types of smokers. Journal of Smoking-Related Disease 5 (suppl 1):179–182, 1994

Fowler JS: Brain monoamine oxidase: an inhibition in cigarette smokers. Proc Natl Acad Sci U S A 93:14065–14069, 1996

Freedman R: Linkage of a neurophysiological deficit in schizophrenia to a chromosome 15 locus. Proc Natl Acad Sci U S A 94:587–592, 1997

Fung YK, Schmid MJ, Anderson TM, et al: Effects of nicotine withdrawal on central dopaminergic systems. Pharmacol Biochem Behav 53:635–640, 1996

George TP, Sernyak MJ, Ziedonis DM, et al: Effects of clozapine on smoking in chronic schizophrenic outpatients. J Clin Psychiatry 56:344–346, 1995

Glassman AH: Cigarette smoking: implications for psychiatric illness. Am J Psychiatry 150:546–553, 1993

Glassman AH: Cigarette Smoking and Its Comorbidity. NIDA Monograph Series No 97-4172. Rockville, MD, U.S. Department of Health and Human Services, 1997

Glassman AH, Stetner F, Walsh Raizman PS, et al: Heavy smokers, smoking cessation, and clonidine: results of a double-blind, randomized trial. JAMA 259:2863–2866, 1988

Glassman AH, Helzer JE, Covey LS, et al: Smoking, smoking cessation and major depression. JAMA 264:1546–1549, 1990

Goff DS, Henderson DC, Amico E: Cigarette smoking in schizophrenia: relationship to psychopathology and medication side effects. Am J Psychiatry 149:1189–1194, 1992

Goldstein MG: Treatment of patients with nicotine dependence. Abstracts of Clinical Care Guidelines 9:23, 1997

Goldstein MG, Niaura R, Abrams DB: Pharmacological and behavioral treatment of nicotine dependence: nicotine as a drug of abuse, in Medical Psychiatric Practice, Vol 1. Edited by Stoudemire A, Fogel BS. Washington, DC, U.S. Government Printing Office, 1991, pp 541–595

Gourlay S: A placebo-controlled study of three clonidine doses for smoking cessation. Clin Pharmacol Ther 55:64–69, 1994

Hall SM, Munoz RF, Reus VI, et al: Nicotine, negative affect and depression. J Consult Clin Psychol 61:761–767, 1993

Hall SM, Munoz RF, Reus VI: Cognitive-behavioral intervention increases abstinence rates for depressive history smokers. J Consult Clin Psychol 62:141–146, 1994

Heatherton T, Kozlowski L, Frecker R, et al: The Fagerstrom test for nicotine dependence: a revision of the Fagerstrom Tolerance Questionnaire. British Journal of Addictions 86:1119–1127, 1991

Henningfield JE, Miyasato K, Jasinski DR: Abuse liability and pharmacodynamic characteristics of intravenous and inhaled nicotine. J Pharmacol Exp Ther 234:1–12, 1985

Hilleman DE: Comparison of fixed-dose transdermal nicotine, tapered-dose transdermal nicotine, and buspirone in smoking cessation. J Clin Pharmacol 34:222–224, 1994

Hoffman AL, Slade J: Addressing tobacco in chemical dependency treatment. J Subst Abuse Treat 10:153–160, 1993

Hughes JR: Prevalence of smoking among psychiatric outpatients. Am J Psychiatry 143:993–997, 1986

Hughes JR: Pharmacotherapy for smoking cessation: unvalidated assumptions, anomalies, and suggestions for future research. J Consult Clin Psychol 61:751–760, 1993

Humfleet G, Hall S, Reus V, et al: The efficacy of nortriptyline as an adjunct to psychological treatment for smokers with and without depressive histories, in Problems of Drug Dependence 1995: Proceedings of the 57th Annual Scientific Meeting, NIDA Research Monograph, Vol 162. Edited by Harris LS. Rockville, MD, National Institute on Drug Abuse, 1996, p 334

Hurt RD: Mortality following inpatient addictions treatment. JAMA 275:1097–1103, 1996

Hurt RD: A comparison of sustained-release bupropion and placebo for smoking cessation. N Engl J Med 337:1195–1202, 1997

Jarvik ME: Beneficial effects of nicotine. British Journal of Addictions 86:571–575, 1991

Keeley EC, Pirwitz MJ, Landau C, et al: Intranasal nicotine spray does not augment the adverse effects of cigarette smoking on myocardial oxygen demand or coronary arterial dimensions. Am J Med 101:357–363, 1996

Kendler KS: Smoking and major depression. Arch Gen Psychiatry 50:36–43, 1993

Kornitzer M: Combined use of nicotine patch and gum in smoking cessation: a placebo-controlled clinical trial. Prev Med 24:41–47, 1995

Law M, Tang JL: An analysis of the effectiveness of interventions intended to help people stop smoking. Arch Intern Med 155:1933–1941, 1995

Leonard S: Nicotinic receptor function in schizophrenia. Schizophr Bull 22:431–445, 1996

Levin ED: Nicotinic systems and cognitive function. Psychopharmacology 108:417–431, 1992

Malin DH, Lake JR, Carter VA, et al: The nicotinic antagonist mecamylamine precipitates nicotine abstinence syndrome in the rat. Psychopharmacology 115:180–184, 1994

McEvoy JP, Freudenrich O, McGee M, et al: Clozapine decreases smoking in patients with chronic schizophrenia. Biol Psychiatry 37:550–552, 1995

McGinnis JM, Foege WH: Actual causes of death in the United States. JAMA 270:2207–2212, 1993

Nides M: Oral presentation at the Society for Research on Nicotine and Tobacco (SRNT), Nashville, TN, June 13, 1997

Olincy A, Young DA, Freedman R: Increased levels of the nicotine metabolite cotinine in schizophrenic smokers compared to other smokers. Biol Psychiatry 42:1–5, 1997

Orleans CT, Slade J (eds): Nicotine Addiction: Principles and Management. Oxford, England, Oxford University Press, 1993

Perkins KA: Acute reinforcing effects of low-dose nicotine nasal spray in humans. Pharmacol Biochem Behav 56:235–241, 1997

Peto R: Mortality from smoking in developed countries 1950–2000. Oxford, England, Oxford University Press, 1994

Pickworth WB: Transdermal nicotine: reduction of smoking with minimal abuse liability. Psychopharmacology 115:9–14, 1994

Pierce JP: Trends in smoking in the United States: projections to the year 2000. JAMA 261:61–65, 1989

Pomerleau OF, Pomerleau CS: Neuroregulators and the reinforcement of smoking: towards a biobehavioral explanation. Neurosci Biobehav Rev 8:503–513, 1984

Pontieri FE, Tanda G, Orzi F, et al: Effects of nicotine on the nucleus accumbens and similarity to those of addictive drugs. Nature 382:255–257, 1996

Prochaska JO, DiClemente CC: Stages of change in the modification of problem behaviors. Prog Behav Modif 28:183–218, 1992

Prochaska JO, Goldstein MG: Process of smoking cessation: implications for clinicians. Clin Chest Med 12:727–735, 1991

Puska P: Is combined use of nicotine patch and gum better than gum alone in smoking cessation? Tobacco Control 4:231–235, 1995

Rose JE, Behm FM, Westman EC, et al: Mecamylamine combined with nicotine skin patch facilitates smoking cessation beyond nicotine patch treatment alone. Clin Pharmacol Ther 56:86–99, 1994

Schneider NG: Efficacy of a nicotine nasal spray in smoking cessation: a placebo-controlled, double-blind trial. Addiction 90:1671–1682, 1995

Schneider NG: Efficacy of buspirone in smoking cessation: a placebo-controlled trial. Clin Pharmacol Ther 60:568–575, 1996a

Schneider NG: Efficacy of a nicotine inhaler in smoking cessation: a double-blind, placebo-controlled trial. Addiction 91:1293–1306, 1996b

Schuh KJ: Nicotine nasal spray and vapor inhaler: abuse liability assessment. Psychopharmacology 130:352–361, 1997

Shiffman SM: Relapse following smoking cessation: a situational analysis. J Consult Clin Psychol 50:71–86, 1982

U.S. Department of Health and Human Services: The Health Consequences of Smoking: Nicotine Addiction. A Report of the Surgeon General. DHHS Pub No CDC-88-8406. Rockville, MD, Office on Smoking and Health, 1988

U.S. Department of Health and Human Services: Clinical Practice Guideline No 18: Smoking Cessation. Washington, DC, U.S. Government Printing Office, 1996

U.S. Preventive Services Task Force: Counseling to prevent tobacco use, in Guide to Clinical Preventive Services, 2nd Edition. Baltimore, MD, Williams & Wilkins, 1996, pp 597–609, 877

Ward KD, Garvey AJ, Bliss RE, et al: Changes in urinary catecholamine excretion after smoking cessation. Pharmacol Biochem Behav 40:937–940, 1991

Warner KE, Slade J, Sweanor DT: The emerging market for long-term nicotine maintenance. JAMA 278:1087–1092, 1997

Zelman D, Brandon T, Jorenby D, et al: Measures of affect and nicotine dependence predict differential response to smoking cessation treatments. J Consult Clin Psychol 60:943–952, 1992

Ziedonis DM, George TP: Schizophrenia and nicotine use: report of a pilot smoking cessation program and review of neurobiological and clinical issues. Schizophr Bull 23(2):247–254, 1997

Ziedonis DM, Kosten TR, Glazer WM, et al: Nicotine dependence and schizophrenia. Hosp Community Psychiatry 45:204–206, 1994

Chapter 2

Alcohol Dependence: Women, Biology, and Pharmacotherapy

Myroslava K. Romach, M.Sc., M.D., F.R.C.P.C., and
Edward M. Sellers, M.D., Ph.D., F.R.C.P.C.

Alcohol use disorders in women are an important public health issue that requires a great deal more attention than it receives. Fifty-nine percent of females drink alcohol; 6% of women have two or more drinks per day, and of these, 15% go on to develop alcohol dependence as defined by DSM-IV (American Psychiatric Association 1994; Wilsnack et al. 1994). Women achieve higher blood alcohol concentrations (BACs) per standard drink than men; are more sensitive to the hepatic, cardiac, and central nervous system complications of chronic alcohol use; and have a more rapid progression of these organic complications. Women's drinking behaviors are also quite different from those of men. With respect to treatment, women use, need, and prefer different services.

Unfortunately, despite considerable progress in the past decade, there exist large gaps in our knowledge about these problems in women. For example, over the past 15 years, a variety of medications have been tested in clinical trials as potential treatments for alcohol dependence, yet from this experience virtually nothing is known about whether these medications are acceptable to women, whether they are effective, and whether alternative treatment approaches may be less costly.

In this chapter, the term *sex* is used to denote biological differences between males and females; *gender* refers to role, behavior, and cognitive differences that represent the consequence of the interaction of sex with environment.

Women's roles in society have undergone rapid and extensive changes in the past 50 years without much evidence that this has been accompanied by equivalent changes in drinking patterns. Examination of the trends and patterns in the general population in North America shows that women continue to remain less likely to drink, to drink less frequently or less heavily, and to report fewer alcohol-related problems than men. These data challenge the hypothesized convergence of men's and women's drinking patterns (L. D. Johnson et al. 1994; Midanik and Clark 1994; Neve et al. 1996; Perkins 1992). Any observed declines in the size of gender differences have resulted mainly from decreases in men's drinking rather than increases in women's drinking (L. D. Johnson et al. 1994; Midanik and Clark 1994). Women's drinking patterns differ according to age, employment and marital status, and ethnicity, as well as a number of other factors. Men generally are more likely to be affected by alcohol use disorders. The male-to-female ratio of lifetime prevalence estimates vary from 2.3:1 for younger adults (age 18–29) (Kessler et al. 1994) to 4–9:1 in older age groups.

Identifying the factors that account for the gender difference in prevalence rates has been difficult. Alcoholism in men and women is determined to some degree by genetic factors, but the contribution of genetic factors alone and their interaction with environmental factors in women are only beginning to be reported. How age, ethnicity, psychiatric comorbidity, and other personal characteristics influence these genetic determinants is incompletely understood. The neurobiological factors that may be transmitted may be expressed as differences in temperament, such as impulsivity, or may be reflected in higher levels of tonic autonomic arousal or increased response to environmental stressors. Vulnerability to other psychiatric illness may also influence risk to development of alcoholism; clinical and epidemiological samples have consistently demonstrated elevated rates of depressive symptoms and of current and lifetime diagnoses of major depression in alcohol-dependent individuals, especially in women (Merikangas and Gelernter 1990; Ross et al. 1988a, 1988b). The capacity to metabolize alcohol may contribute to differences in prevalence rates; women exhibit reduced levels of alcohol dehydrogenase (ADH) in the stomach, leading to slightly higher levels of alcohol in the blood. Gender differences in subjective and behavioral responses to alcohol that increase risk for alcoholism may also be genetically mediated. At present, gender differences in alcohol use remain largely unexplained. Any explanation will need to be multidimensional and will have to examine the interaction of biological, personal, and sociocultural differences.

The goal of this chapter is to summarize the evidence indicating that women, ethanol, and the environment interact in ways that should determine that public health and health services policies and practice specifically address the unique needs of women. Our perspective is focused on the biological aspects of alcohol use and how medications may be developed and used as adjuncts in the treatment of alcohol dependence.

Physiological Differences

Numerous reviews of ethanol metabolism and disposition exist and can be consulted for a general background overview (Lieber 1997; Thomasson 1995). Body size, composition, gastric emptying rate, presence of concurrent food, food composition, smoking status, ethanol concentration in beverage, beverage type, gastric and hepatic blood flow, quantitative and qualitative differences in alcohol-metabolizing enzymes, diurnal physiological variations, total and relative body water, and sex have all been shown to affect ethanol disposition (Lieber 1997).

Volume of Distribution

BACs in women are higher than in men after consuming the same amount of alcohol because women weigh less than men and have a slightly lower total body water content per body mass, which is associated with a higher relative fat content (Lieber 1997; Thomasson 1995). Reported volumes of distribution for ethanol are 18%–26% smaller in women. Therefore, to the extent that alcoholic beverages are dispensed and ingested in standard "doses," women are at greater risk for intoxication than are men. However, because ethanol is primarily consumed and titrated by the individual for its reinforcing properties while balancing against aversive effects, the rate and amount of alcohol ingested are likely to be less in women than men as long as sensitivity is equal. In most clinical studies, women typically consume about 20% less alcohol than men, which coincides fairly closely with the expected differences in BACs after a standard drink. When women receive the same dose of ethanol based on volume of distribution corrected for body weight, mean BAC does not differ from that of men. Although total body water may vary during the phases of the menstrual cycle, these changes do not appear to alter BACs when ethanol is administered in a dose corrected for volume of distribution (Brick et al. 1986).

Biotransformation

In addition to the prominent effect of differences in volume of distribution on ethanol disposition in women as compared with men, there appear to be large inter- and intraindividual variations in metabolic capacity, or intrinsic metabolic clearance for ethanol. Alcohol is eliminated primarily by ADH, cytochrome P450 enzymes (e.g., cytochrome P450 2E1 [CYP2E1]), and catalase. ADH exists in five isoforms with different activities. These are not sex linked, and they show important ethnoracial variations (Lieber 1997). ADH is quantitatively the most important enzyme but has a low affinity for ethanol. In contrast, CYP2E1 has a higher affinity for ethanol but a lower capacity. CYP2E1 is found in the liver and brain, is inducible by alcohol and other drugs, and during metabolism can produce tissue-damaging free radicals from ethanol and other drugs (e.g., acetaminophen, even at therapeutic doses).

The published literature concerning male-female differences in ethanol metabolism must be viewed with caution because of important differences in study designs. Of 12 published studies, 6 (one including 400 sets of twins) failed to find a sex difference in metabolism (Thomasson et al. 1994); 5 showed that women have faster ethanol metabolic rates of elimination than men; and 4 others showed numerically larger, but not significantly different, clearances. Among the significant studies, the women had a terminal elimination rate that was 28% more rapid than that in men, but in three of these studies the differences in rate were not significant once corrected for body weight and volume of distribution.

The reasons for faster elimination of ethanol in women are not clear because there is no evidence that the amounts of the enzymes responsible for metabolizing ethanol (ADH, catalase, CYP2E1) are constitutively expressed at different levels in females and males. Sex differences in the amount of hepatic ADH have been shown in rodents, but rodents are notorious for showing sexual dimorphisms in drug metabolism. If human CYP2E1 messenger RNA expression, stability, translation, and protein degradation were shown to be affected by sex hormones, CYP2E1 would be a prime candidate to explain the differential rates of ethanol metabolism in some females and would provide an explanation for the increased risk of hepatic and brain damage in women.

Sex hormone effects on ethanol metabolism. Lammers et al. (1995) reviewed studies of the effect of the menstrual cycle on ethanol kinetics. Of 11 published studies, only 2 met their stringent criteria for validity. Both of these studies showed significantly faster elimination of alcohol during the luteal phase (days 23–28) of the menstrual cycle. The elimination rate of alcohol was about 14% higher during the luteal phase than during all other phases of the cycle. Progesterone levels are also highest in the luteal phase, suggesting an impact of this hormone on ethanol metabolism; therefore, progesterone-containing medications might also modestly increase ethanol elimination.

Does this faster elimination rate have any behavioral or physiological implications? The small difference detected in a 4- to 5-day phase under stringent test conditions compared with all other sources of within- and between-female differences suggests that it is only a kinetic curiosity. During some days of the menstrual cycle, some women may experience slightly lower BACs than usual, but, at least based on available data, this will occur only in normally cycling females during ovulatory cycles. In many women this phenomenon will not apply or may not occur (Lammers et al. 1995). Because heavy chronic drinking can cause anovulation and other sex hormone changes, it is questionable whether these kinetic changes apply to women with alcohol abuse or dependence.

The complex interaction of drinking pattern, race, body composition, age, and sex steroid levels across time offers a challenging research opportunity. To date, there are no convincing data that the human female menstrual cycle importantly alters ethanol kinetics and accounts for more variable ethanol effects in women than men.

First-pass metabolism. Some women have a smaller first-pass metabolism of alcohol than men due to lesser amounts of ADH in the stomach and upper small intestine, which metabolize alcohol en route to the liver. This results in higher systemic bioavailability of ethanol (Lieber 1997). Because the absolute amounts of enzyme in the stomach and gut are low, the impact of this first-pass metabolism is greatest at low ethanol doses. However, the clinical importance of this phenomenon is controversial. Frezza et al. (1990) initially showed that Italian nonalcoholic women had about one-quarter and alcoholic women one-eighth the first-pass metabolism of ethanol relative to men, and that women's gastric ADH content was 60% that of men's. Other investigations have not confirmed this finding in other ethnoracial groups (Ammon et al. 1996). Some differences in ADH-specific isoform expression in gastric tissue in women and men may account for these different results. A recent study in Germans, in which oral and intraduodenal deuterated ethanol and intravenous ethanol were used, revealed that first-pass gastric metabolism in males and females after low ethanol dose (0.3 g/kg) was small (9.1% and 8.4%, respectively) and was only partly of gastric origin (Ammon et al. 1996).

Susceptibility to Organic Damage

Women are more sensitive than men to the organic complications of alcohol on the liver, heart, and brain. For most alcohol-associated disorders (e.g., fatty liver, hypertension, obesity, anemia, malnutrition, gastrointestinal hemorrhage, and ulcers requiring surgery [Van Thiel et al. 1989]), women have had lower total lifetime exposure to ethanol at time of assessment.

Liver. The risk of developing liver damage is greater in women than men for both lower and identical patterns of consumption (Van Thiel et al. 1989). In addition, once women develop alcoholic hepatitis, the rate of progression is faster than in men (i.e., a "telescoping" effect on the time frame of disease progression). As a result, when the problem is recognized in women, liver damage is often more advanced, and the prognosis much worse, than in men. Of those who continue to drink once a diagnosis has been made, only 30% of women, compared with 72% of men, survive for 5 years. When women die, they are 11 years younger on average then men. Even among those who stop or reduce alcohol intake, alcoholic hepatitis progresses in 50% of women but rarely in men under the same conditions (Deal and Gavaler 1994).

Heart. The female heart also seems to be more sensitive to the adverse effects of ethanol. An epidemiological study indicated that, despite a 40% lower lifetime exposure to alcohol in women, the decline in cardiac function that occurs is similar to that in men (Urbano-Márquez et al. 1995). In addition, the slope relating total lifetime dose of alcohol to left ventricular ejection fraction is significantly more negative in women than in men, indicating greater sensitivity to damage.

Brain. The data are not clear concerning organic brain damage in women as compared with men; however, neuropsychological function is impaired to a greater extent for equivalent alcohol intake in women, as evidenced by greater widening of cerebral sulci and fissures (Mann et al. 1992). Women exhibit abnormalities on computerized tomography of the brain after a shorter drinking history and at lower peak alcohol consumption. Women also perform less well on psychological tests of recall, speech, and perceptual accuracy, despite a less severe drinking history than that of men.

Ethanol Effects on Sex Hormones

Alcohol consumption alters the balance of circulating reproductive hormones in women. Acute administration of alcohol to premenopausal women results in an increase in plasma estradiol in the follicular and luteal phases (Mendelson et al. 1988). Similarly, in postmenopausal women wearing estradiol skin patches (Ginsburg et al. 1995) or taking oral micronized estrogen replacement therapy, acute alcohol administration leads to significantly increased levels of estradiol, probably due in part to decreases in estradiol metabolism (Ginsburg et al. 1996). As estrogen replacement therapy becomes more common, women who drink alcohol may have significantly higher estradiol levels than expected.

Several groups have studied the effect of chronic alcohol consumption on various sex hormone concentrations (Dorgan et al. 1994; Harris et al. 1995). The main effects of alcohol across cycle phases in premenopausal women are to increase plasma dehydroepiandrosterone (follicular and luteal phases) and estrone (ovulatory phase) and increase urinary estradiol (ovulatory and luteal phases) and estrone (luteal phase). Dorgan et al. (1994) found that alcohol increased average plasma levels of androstenedione in premenopausal women. Alcohol can increase luteinizing hormone production, which in turn stimulates ovarian thecal cells to secrete androstenedione. This compound, in turn, is metabolized to estrone and estradiol by ovarian granulosa cells in response to follicle-stimulating hormone, which has been hypothesized to be inhibited by alcohol (Mello 1980). Chronic heavy sustained alcohol use leads to menstrual dysfunction, spontaneous abortion, and amenorrhea (Hugues et al. 1980; Moskovic 1975) in premenopausal women. Chronic alcohol ingestion increases estradiol concentrations by decreasing its metabolism, possibly by the liver cytochromes CYP1A2, CYP3A, or CYP2E1.

Hepatic dysfunction resulting from alcoholism itself leads to disturbances in the menstrual cycle and earlier menopause. Postmenopausal women with chronic liver disease have significant disturbances of sex hormone metabolism with elevated estrone levels (Becker 1993).

The clinical implications of these various (and sometimes small) hormonal changes under various conditions of ethanol ingestion are not known. Apart from the effects of heavy chronic ingestion, which causes anovulation, few clinically important consequences have been identified in premenopausal women. Several interesting studies in postmenopausal women have suggested that the hormonal changes can be important. Post-menopausal women who drink at least 7 ounces (210 ml) of ethanol per week have significantly higher bone density (7.7%) than women drinking less than 1 ounce (30 ml) per week, an effect that is possibly related to the augmentation of endogenous estrogen levels by alcohol (Felson et al. 1995). Higher estradiol levels are associated with decreased risks of osteoporosis and coronary artery disease. However, epidemiological studies have shown that alcohol ingestion increases the risk of breast cancer in post-menopausal and possibly premenopausal women (Dorgan et al. 1994). Changes in blood levels of estrogens and androgens have been proposed as a possible explanation. In the light of the increasing number of women using some form of estrogen replacement therapy in North America, the potential health risks and benefits of the interactions between alcohol and hormone replacement therapy need to be evaluated further.

Behavioral Pharmacology: Gender Differences in Alcohol Effects

Table 2–1 summarizes studies that have examined differences in behavioral responses to ethanol between males and females. Interpretation of these studies is difficult. Variations in dose, methods of ethanol administration, dependent variable selection and methodology, and testing times are rarely comparable. It is important that failure to characterize the within- and between-subject and day-to-day variation in response and to generate within-subject dose-response data severely weaken the power of the published data.

The strongest evidence for sex differences comes from cognitive research, which suggests that such effects have complex interactions with dose, expectancy, and ethanol concentration. This is not unexpected because gender differences in cognitive abilities and cerebral lateralization have been reported for many years (Drake et al. 1990). These types of studies are difficult to perform, and few have been done. This is an area in which more extensive human laboratory research could be particularly useful.

Table 2–1.   Summary of reports comparing effects of ethanol in females and males[a]

Reference	Result	Comment
Jones and Jones 1976	Females were more impaired than males on delayed, but not immediate recall memory.	Females had higher BACs because the ethanol dose was not adjusted for body weight.
Burns and Moskowitz 1978	No differences were found between males and females in hand steadiness, body sway, response latency, or information processing.	No BAC or kinetic differences were found, despite identical dose/body weight.
Taberner 1980	A complex interaction was found among dose, sex, and time of testing on simple reaction time. At a high ethanol dose (0.76 ml/kg), females showed significant impairment only toward the end of testing, whereas males demonstrated increased response latencies throughout testing (30–90 min).	Despite ethanol being given on a body weight basis, no differences in BAC were found.
Sutker et al. 1982	No female/male differences were found on physiological arousal, subjective distress after threat of electric shock, subjective intoxication, or BAC.	A complex interaction was found among beverage consumed, expectancy, and gender on measured anxiety.

Wait et al. 1982	No female/male differences were found on measures of mirror tracing, dart throwing, or perceived high or pleasantness. Males were more variable than females on prism adaptation and a pointing task.	Alcohol doses (1.25 g/kg) were identical in the groups. BAC data were not reported.
Mills and Bisgrove 1983	No female/male differences were found on body sway at any of three ethanol doses (0, 0.37, and 0.76 g/kg). At higher doses, females were more impaired on divided attention than males.	Females perceived themselves to be significantly less impaired. Alcohol doses were adjusted for percent body fat; hence, females achieved BACs at lower doses that were similar to those achieved by males at higher doses.
Niaura et al. 1987	Males recovered memory function more quickly than females on the descending side of the BAC curve after dose (0.65 g/kg) was corrected for BAC differences. No differences were seen on divided attention, body sway, pursuit tracking, or subjective level of intoxication.	BACs were higher in middle stage of menstrual cycle. Menstrual cycle phase did not influence psychomotor or cognitive performance in women.
Lex et al. 1988	Females with negative family history showed significantly more errors on the DSST and body sway effects than females with positive family history. Compared with literature controls, both groups reported less intoxication than men.	Study compared females with positive and negative family histories, with no male control group.

(continued)

Table 2-1. Summary of reports comparing effects of ethanol in females and males [a] *(continued)*

Reference	Result	Comment
Ammon et al. 1996	A linear relationship was found between BAC and a sedation index. The slope of the regression line was steeper in females (1.04) than in males (0.42).	Data were pooled from several test sessions, and the overall regression, although significant ($P < .001$), was weak: $r = .34$ (males) and .65 (females).
Acker 1985	Alcoholic females performed significantly less well than matched nonalcoholic control subjects on neuropsychological tests. The deficits were similar to those reported for males, despite significantly shorter drinking histories.	
Ciraulo et al. 1996	Daughters of alcoholic persons ($n = 12$) had greater pleasant mood responses than a control group ($n = 11$) after a single dose (1 mg) of alprazolam. Daughters of alcoholic persons also showed lower self-esteem and satisfaction with the rest of the world than did control subjects.	The differences in abuse liability measures in the daughters of alcoholic persons from the control group were surprisingly large, despite apparent matching on actual and past drug use.
George et al. 1997	Type I alcoholic subjects reported more anger and anxiety after mCPP (a non-selective serotonergic agonist that can induce craving in alcohol-dependent individuals), whereas type II alcoholic subjects reported increased euphoria and a greater likelihood of drinking.	This study was done only in males. How-ever, type II alcoholic individuals are more likely to be early-onset, more severely affected males with a paternal history of alcohol and antisocial behavior. An equivalent study in females might be expected to show more of the type I re-

de Wit and Chutuape 1993	Ingestion of a moderate dose (0.25–0.5 g/kg) of ethanol increased the tendency to continue drinking, even among normal drinkers (19 males, 9 females). No mean gender differences were reported; however, more males than females (75% vs. 50%; NS) chose to continue drinking after the primary dose.	sponse because negative mood states appear to play a more important role for women. Ethanol dose was not corrected for volume of distribution/body weight. BACs were not reported. Chooser/nonchooser (to keep drinking) status may have been affected by interaction of subjective response with ethanol kinetics.
Davidson et al. 1997	Subjects (7 males and 8 females) were unable to report positive alcohol effects until the ascending side of an infusion achieved a BAC of 40 mg/dl. No gender differences were reported.	Ethanol was administered intravenously based on a nomogram to compensate for sex, height, weight, and age to yield target BACs of 0, 10, 20, and 40 mg/dl. The sensitivity of the subjective measures may not have been sufficient.
Drake et al. 1990	Male but not female chronic alcoholic subjects exhibited right-hemisphere dysfunction. Females, alcoholic or not, appeared to be less lateralized in function.	In contrast to other studies, females did not appear to be as vulnerable to the effects of chronic alcohol abuse. In females (and males), there was some suggestion of a decrease in intellectual function, but in females no alcohol-related changes were noted in hemispheric asymmetry of function.

[a] BAC = blood alcohol concentration; DSST = Digit Symbol Substitution Test; mCPP = *m*-chlorophenylpiperazine; NS = not significant.

Alcohol Dependence and Psychiatric Comorbidity

Data from the National Institute of Mental Health Epidemiologic Catchment Area (ECA) Study (Reiger et al. 1990) indicated that 37% of alcohol-abusing individuals met DSM-III-R (American Psychiatric Association 1987) criteria for at least one other psychiatric disorder. In a recent Canadian study, the Ontario Health Survey (Ross 1995), 55% of individuals with an alcohol disorder had a lifetime history of a comorbid psychiatric disorder, and this comorbidity was more common in women than men. These individuals had a significantly increased risk of mood and anxiety disorders than did respondents without an alcohol disorder. Comorbidity may alter the time of onset and clinical course of alcoholism, affect the therapeutic intervention selected, and alter treatment outcome, and there may be gender differences in these variables (Rounsaville et al. 1987). Negative affective states such as anxiety and depression appear to initiate and maintain maladaptive drinking patterns (Marlatt and Gordon 1985) and may be important in relapse to drinking (Litt et al. 1990). Alleviation of these dysphoric states, pharmacologically or psychologically, could lead to a decrease in or cessation of excessive drinking.

Self-Medication Hypothesis

The public, clinicians, and patients commonly believe that one of the reasons individuals drink is because alcohol reduces anxiety and tension and alleviates low mood. Such a belief has clinical appeal because it offers a rather straightforward explanation for the etiology of alcohol use problems: Anxious and depressed individuals drink alcohol to relieve their symptoms, and this self-medication turns into problematic use. However, it has proven extremely difficult to substantiate this process with empirical data, and it is based primarily on anecdotal reports.

Liebenluft et al. (1993) examined the relationship between depressive symptoms and the self-reported use of alcohol in normal volunteers and four groups of psychiatric outpatients, 75% of them female. They found that for each depressive symptom examined, the alcohol-dependent patients were more likely than non–alcohol-dependent patients to drink in response to that symptom and were more likely than the other patients to report that alcohol relieved each of the depressive symptoms. Among alcohol-dependent subjects, those without major depression were as likely as those with comorbid depression to report drinking in response to depressive symptoms. In addition, alcohol-dependent subjects could be distinguished from other subjects by the degree to which they reported that drinking relieved anger and social anxiety.

Most of the studies exploring the interaction between alcohol and mood have concentrated on the relationship between alcohol consumption and the behavioral and psychological responses to stressful stimuli (Cappell and Greeley 1987). As a result, there has been a greater emphasis in the human experimental and clinical literature on the effects of alcohol on anxious rather than depressive affect. Much of the research investigating the extent to which alcohol consumption is motivated by the intent of "tension" reduction is experimental in nature.

Human experimental studies have shown that alcohol in modest doses reduces levels of anxiety in laboratory paradigms of performance anxiety in normal subjects (Mayfield 1979). However, the experimental methods and measures used have been extremely heterogeneous; most of these studies used volunteer subjects without clinically significant anxiety, and this has resulted in conflicting results. Variables that determine the effects of alcohol on anxiety include the amount of alcohol consumed and individual physiological differences that influence response to alcohol, including steroidal hormones in women, previous experiences with alcohol, expectations about the effects of alcohol, cognitive set, gender, and how anxiety is defined. In an excellent review of this area, Wilson (1988) argued that the more relevant question is "At what dose, under which conditions, in whom, and on what measures does alcohol reduce anxiety?" (p. 371).

Despite the conflicting and often inconclusive data reported in support of self-medication or tension reduction as a primary motivating factor in the initiation and maintenance of drinking behavior, this hypothesis continues to be of great clinical interest and is often referred to when attempts are made to account for the high rates of comorbidity of alcohol disorders and other psychiatric illnesses.

Outcome Expectancies

The beliefs and expectations that individuals have about the effects of alcohol and the consequences of drinking may influence drinking patterns and related behavioral responses to alcohol and may account for some of the published data describing self-medication of negative affective states. Goldman et al. (1987) have shown that expectations about the stress-reducing effects of alcohol are correlated with drinking behavior in different populations and that alcohol-related beliefs may interact with the pharmacological properties of alcohol to determine intoxication experiences (Abrams and Niaura 1987). It has been reported that, in general, women and men respond differently to the expectancy that alcohol has been consumed, particularly in situations of social interaction, suggesting a gender difference in the content of alcohol-related expectancies (Sutker et al. 1982). In social interaction paradigms, the belief that alcohol has been consumed results in a reduction of self-reported anxiety in males, whereas females more often, but not always (de Boer et al. 1993), respond with an increase in anxiety. Women appear to expect less positive and more negative effects from alcohol than men—more cognitive and physical impairment and disinhibition (Gustafson 1991). Part of this difference may be due to the fact that men and women have different direct and indirect past experiences with alcohol. Leigh (1989) has proposed that the same alcohol outcome expectancies could lead to different behaviors depending on the salience of the expected outcome in a particular situation. Perhaps women facing anxiety-provoking situations associate the tension-reducing effects of alcohol with loss of control and increased vulnerability, whereas men may value the reduced inhibitions and diminished sense of responsibility associated with the anxiolytic effects of alcohol (Kushner et al. 1994).

Published data on expectancies of tension reduction and effects on alcohol consumption have not always been consistent. Corcoran and Parker (1991) found that the belief that alcohol reduces tension did not always predict alcohol consumption in a stressful situation in normal volunteers. Most reports are based on experimental studies, and individuals' alcohol expectancies and responses to alcohol in a laboratory setting may be different from those in a natural drinking situation (Sher 1985). The significance of the relationship between alcohol problems and beliefs about tension reduction in clinical populations, however, has been confirmed. Brown (1985) found that beliefs about tension reduction were important predictors of relapse after treatment. Expectancies about the tension-reducing effects of alcohol among untreated problem drinkers are stronger than those among nonproblem drinkers and are significantly altered after successful treatment of the drinking problems (Young and Longmore 1987). Cox et al. (1993) found that male patients who had panic disorder with agoraphobia were more likely to perceive alcohol as an effective strategy in coping with anxiety and reported more weekly alcohol intake than did female patients.

From the existing data, it would appear that the interaction of pharmacology, expectancy of outcome, gender role, situation, and affective state, as they relate to tension reduction or self-medication, is important in understanding the drinking behavior of many, although not all, individuals.

Depression and Alcohol Dependence

In the epidemiological studies cited above, individuals with a lifetime diagnosis of alcohol abuse and/or dependence consistently have an increased risk for major depression; relative risks range from 1.5 to 4.5 (Grant and Harford 1995; Merikangas and Gelernter 1990; Reiger et al. 1990). In a recently completed, 12-week, controlled clinical trial of dexfenfluramine versus placebo, 34% of alcoholic patients presenting for treatment had a lifetime history of major depression, as determined with a validated structured diagnostic interview (Structured Clinical Interview for DSM-III-R Diagnoses [SCID]), and extensive depressive symptomatology irrespective of diagnostic category (Romach et al. 1995). Depression is a serious disorder accompanied by significant distress and disability (von Korff et al. 1992) and an increased risk (10%–15%) of suicide completion in alcoholism (Schuckit 1986).

Although it has been traditional to classify depression with diagnostic approaches and to separate depression in alcoholism into primary and secondary types (Schuckit 1986), this temporal convenience of classification fails to account for the complex and intertwined nature of mood disorders with the drinking behavior and largely ignores the observation that the "diagnosis" of major depression seems to have little to do with symptoms and function (Gotlieb et al. 1995). Although conceptually attractive, a causal or self-medication model to account for the comorbidity between depression and alcoholism is difficult to evaluate rigorously. Some information about the plausibility of this model is provided by evaluating the ages at onset of the two conditions in comorbid cases. The ECA study found that for those individuals with a diagnosis of both major depression and alcoholism, 66% of women reported that major depression was the antecedent diagnosis, whereas most men stated that their depression developed after the alcohol problems (Helzer and Pryzbeck 1988). Kendler et al. (1993) reported similar results in that 63% of women with comorbid diagnoses in their entirely female sample had the onset of major depression before the onset of alcohol dependence. Gorman (1992) has argued that subclinical episodes of depression frequently precede the onset of alcohol problems and should also be assessed as possible predisposing factors in the development of alcohol dependence.

Depressed mood has been hypothesized to play a more prominent role in the drinking behavior of women (Turnbull and Gomberg 1988), although much of what is known about psychopathology and alcoholism is derived from studies of men (Penick et al. 1988). Alcohol-abusing women are as much as four times more likely than men to complain of depressive symptoms (Jaffe and Ciraulo 1986). Women more often report that depressive symptoms accompany their drinking problems and that depression preceded the onset of their alcohol problems (A. T. Beck et al. 1982; Hatsukami and Pickens 1982). Turnbull and Gomberg (1990) reported that in a sample of 301 alcoholic women asked about events that brought them into treatment, the largest proportion (88%) responded that it was because they were feeling "low" and depressed.

This again raises the question of whether women are more likely to attempt to cope with or to self-medicate feelings of depression by drinking alcohol. Schutte et al. (1995) conducted a 3-year follow-up of depressive symptoms and drinking behavior in a nonclinical group of 621 older men and women. They found that, although higher initial levels of depressive symptoms did not lead to increased alcohol consumption among men or women, heavier initial levels of alcohol consumption were associated with lower levels of depression over the course of 1 and 3 years in women. One interpretation of these results was that alcohol consumption was part of a process related to the successful alleviation of depressive symptoms.

Estrogen has been proposed as one of the modulators for the interaction between depressive symptoms and alcohol intake. Human data indicate that low estrogen levels may be associated with depression (Wheatley 1991). Stress often precedes depression and may in itself reduce estrogen levels (Ballinger 1991). Alcohol may relieve the symptoms of depression, as it is reported to increase serum estradiol levels in women (Gavaler and Van Thiel 1992). Therefore, the common biological denominator that mediates alcoholism and depression in women may be low serum estradiol levels (Hilakivi-Clarke 1996). This interaction could also involve brain serotonergic turnover, as serotonergic receptors and 5-hydroxytryptamine (5-HT [serotonin]) content and turnover are modulated by steroidal hormones (S. G. Beck et al. 1989) in discrete brain nuclei. Diminished or dysregulated 5-HT activity has been linked to alcohol intake and depression (Sellers et al. 1991).

Several studies of treated alcoholic patients suggest that concomitant psychopathology may have different treatment outcome implications for males and females (Kranzler et al. 1992; Rounsaville et al. 1987). Rounsaville et al. (1987) found that alcoholic women who experienced depressive problems had comparatively good posttreatment outcomes on alcohol-related measures as compared with men and with women without depressive problems. However, there is relatively little empirical evidence to support this suggestion.

Pharmacological alleviation of depressive symptoms can have a beneficial effect in decreasing drinking (Cornelius et al. 1997).

In the light of the prevalence of depressive comorbidity in women, the availability of effective antidepressant medications, and studies suggesting that remediation of comorbid depression may improve outcome for drinking problems, it is important for appropriately controlled clinical trials to be conducted in women to determine definitively whether such a strategy provides an enhanced treatment option.

Anxiety and Alcohol Dependence

Similar to the evidence presented for depression, results of clinical and epidemiological studies have consistently shown substantial co-occurrence of anxiety disorders and alcohol problems (Helzer and Pryzbeck 1988; Ross et al. 1988b). Although anxiety disorders are highly prevalent in the general population, the odds ratios indicate that anxiety disorders are risk factors for alcohol problems (Kushner and Sher 1993). The ECA survey reported some gender differences in the association of alcohol abuse and/or dependence and specific anxiety disorders. Among individuals with an alcohol use disorder, women were more than three times as likely as men to have panic disorder and more than twice as likely to have a phobia (Helzer and Pryzbeck 1988).

The nature of the relationship between anxiety disorders and alcohol use is complex, and as with depressive symptoms, there has been much speculation about the functional relevance of anxiety symptoms. For some individuals, anxiety symptoms may be etiologically related to the alcohol disorder, whether by contributing to the initiation of drinking or by predisposing to the return to alcohol use after a period of abstinence as the individual attempts to alleviate symptoms of dysphoria. The various anxiety disorders have different relationships with alcohol problems. Social phobia and agoraphobia tend to precede the development of alcohol disorders, whereas panic disorder and generalized anxiety disorder often follow the onset of alcohol problems and in some patients may be related to alcohol withdrawal.

Yanofsky et al. (1986) have proposed that alcohol does not modify affects such as tension or anxiety directly, but rather does so via changes in cognitive perceptual processing of incoming information. In this way, alcohol decreases self-awareness and hence negative and anxiety-inducing self-evaluation, or it narrows perceptions to the most immediate and salient cues in the environment so that the individual loses the capacity to process information about more distant worries (Steele and Josephs 1988). Such cognitive processes and attributions may differ between men and women and may be differentially affected by alcohol. They also appear to be more relevant in the phobic disorders and may account for the higher rates of comorbidity of agoraphobia and social phobia with alcohol problems.

From a neurobiological perspective, neuroactive steroids may play a role in the interaction of alcohol and anxiety symptoms. Pharmacological and biochemical studies have shown that two specific 5α-reduced metabolites (allopregnanolone) of progesterone possess anxiolytic activity in animal models of anxiety and suggest that the behavioral effects of these metabolites involve interactions with the γ-aminobutyric acid–A (GABA-A) receptor complex (Bitran et al. 1993). Neurosteroids may be responsible, in part, for the observed differences between male and female animals in the response of the GABA system to alcohol.

Animal studies have shown behavioral differences in anxiety across the ovarian cycle in females (Carey et al. 1992). Brot et al. (1995) found that alcohol administered to rats in different phases of the estrous cycle was more effective as an anxiolytic when hormone levels were high. Increased sensitivity to the benzodiazepine triazolam was demonstrated when progesterone was co-administered to postmenopausal women (McAuley et al. 1995). Similar enhanced sensitivity in the presence of elevated progesterone concentrations may occur with other psychoactive substances, including alcohol.

Several studies have explored a possible relationship between alcohol use and premenstrual dysphoria in clinical samples (Belfer and Shader 1976). Retrospective reports found that premenstrual tension was related to increased drinking by alcoholic women and by social drinkers. Prospective studies, however, have not confirmed increased consumption premenstrually in nonalcoholic drinking women (Charette et al. 1990; Sutker et al. 1983).

Clearly more work is required to understand hormonal inter-actions with alcohol consumption and to determine whether the differential effects of alcohol among women as a function of the menstrual cycle are perceptual or pharmacological in origin. With renewed interest in steroidal hormone regulation of mood and anxiety in women, more information will be forthcoming about the role of these compounds in clinical disorders of anxiety, de-pression, and alcohol use.

Treatment Services

Identification of Alcohol Dependence in Women

Health care professionals are less likely to recognize alcohol abuse or dependence in women than in men, and when it is pres-ent, they are less likely to offer the same treatment opportunities as they would to men. In a primary care setting, male patients were 1.5 times more likely than women to have been warned about alcohol use and 3 times more likely to have been told to stop or modify their consumption once they had been identified as "at risk" by a screening questionnaire (Volk et al. 1996).

The underrecognition of alcohol-related problems in women has been attributed to higher psychiatric comorbidity (depression and anxiety disorders) in females than in males. The recognition of specific anxiety disorders and major depression by primary care physicians is not optimal; however, symptoms of these dis-orders may provide a sufficient clinical distraction to create a di-agnostic blindness to the existence of an alcohol use disorder (Volk et al. 1996). Standard methods to screen for and identify alcohol problems may have limited usefulness in women because they are typically directed at detecting severe or advanced stages of alcohol dependence associated with physical dependence, or-ganic complications, and serious psychosocial dysfunction. Dif-ferent approaches need to be developed to identify problem drinking in women (Chan 1993), particularly in the early stages.

Barriers to Treatment

Many authors have suggested that gender differences in service utilization for alcohol abuse may reflect the existence of barriers that specifically affect women (Schober and Annis 1996). Treatment or, more simply, a change in drug use behavior can be conceptualized as a process that is mediated by several interacting factors, including background characteristics (e.g., gender, substance use history), stage of change preparedness, the decision-making process involving health beliefs and appraisals, reasons for change, and offsetting barriers to change (Schober and Annis 1996). Treatment trials for alcohol dependence should take these important issues into account because they are probably responsible for the large variation in female participation in clinical trials and outcome variation between the sexes.

For example, women appear to conceptualize the etiology of their alcohol problem differently than men. Women are more likely than men to identify anxiety, depression, and stressful life events as their main difficulties and to attribute drinking to their attempts to control these experiences (Thom 1986). Women may not seek help in the same way or may delay seeking help because of social practices and policies. For example, women, if identified as having an alcohol problem, are more likely to be regarded as deviant because they diverge from their gender role of child care-givers. A unimodal treatment program structure that does not address these specific needs of women (e.g., availability of sexual and physical abuse counseling, child care, medical and nutritional care, treatment of psychiatric disorders) may discourage women from entering treatment (Schober and Annis 1996).

Medication Development

In the last decade, advances in understanding the neurobiological mechanisms of alcohol abuse and dependence have established that the reinforcing effects of alcohol are mediated by several neurotransmitter systems and endogenous peptides, and that it is their interaction that affects alcohol consumption (e.g., the serotonergic and endogenous opioid systems). Drugs acting on these systems have been the focus of research to develop effective medications for the treatment of alcoholism.

The most extensively studied group of drugs have been those with serotonergic activity. Although initial short-term clinical trials with 5-HT uptake inhibitors showed some promise, for example, with fluoxetine (Naranjo et al. 1990) and citalopram (Naranjo et al. 1987), a larger treatment trial failed to demonstrate the efficacy of fluoxetine in the treatment of alcohol dependence (Kranzler et al. 1995). More specifically acting compounds have also been evaluated. Dexfenfluramine, a 5-HT releaser and uptake inhibitor, was found to be no more effective than placebo in reducing alcohol consumption in alcohol-dependent individuals (Romach et al. 1996). At low doses, ondansetron, a 5-HT, subtype 3 (5-HT$_3$), receptor antagonist, showed some modest reduction in alcohol intake in patients, but not of sufficient magnitude to justify its clinical use (Sellers et al. 1994). Ritanserin, a 5-HT$_2$ receptor antagonist, also has been shown to be ineffective (B. A. Johnson et al. 1996).

Serotonergically acting drugs, however, may be more effective in the treatment of alcohol dependence in patients with concurrent psychiatric illness. A recent double-blind, placebo-controlled trial of fluoxetine in depressed, hospitalized alcoholic patients showed the medication significantly reduced depressive symptoms and total alcohol consumption as compared with placebo (Cornelius et al. 1997). Similarly, positive results have been obtained with other nonserotonergic antidepressants, imipramine (McGrath et al. 1996) and desipramine (Mason et al. 1996), in the treatment of depressed, alcohol-dependent individuals.

In a similar vein, a number of studies have been conducted with buspirone, a 5-HT$_{1A}$ agonist and anxiolytic, in alcohol-dependent patients with and without clinically significant anxiety (Kranzler et al. 1997; Malcolm et al. 1992; Tollefson et al. 1992). The results have been mixed, and clear-cut evidence for the efficacy of buspirone in improving drinking-related outcomes in anxious alcoholic patients is lacking. Mild to moderately impaired patients may find the medication beneficial, particularly if their anxiety symptoms fall within the category of generalized anxiety.

More recently, two different types of medication have generated great clinical interest. The opiate antagonist naltrexone was shown to be useful in the treatment of alcohol dependence in two clinical trials (O'Malley et al. 1992; Volpicelli et al. 1992). The drug was shown to reduce craving and relapse rates in abstinent subjects and amount of alcohol consumption in patients who continued to drink. Other opiate antagonists are also being investigated for their clinical utility (Mason et al. 1994), and possible combinations with other psychotropic drugs may prove useful.

Acamprosate, a structural analogue of homocysteic acid that may interact with excitatory amino acid neurotransmitters, has been tested in Europe. A large multisite trial showed acamprosate to increase the number of abstinent days in alcoholic patients for up to 1 year as compared with placebo (Sass et al. 1996). Trials with this medication are presently under way in the United States.

Medications in Women

Ideally, what is known about sex and gender differences in sensitivity to alcohol's behavioral and organic effects, ethanol disposition, cognitive processes, psychiatric comorbidity, behavioral pharmacology, health service utilization, and preferences would set the medication development research agenda concerning alcohol dependence in women. To assess the extent to which knowledge informs practice, we reviewed all reports of clinical research trials and human experimental studies involving medications for treatment of alcohol dependence for the period from 1980 to October 1997. Our goal was to determine the extent to which women participated in these trials and the extent to which data analysis addressed differences between males and females. We identified a total of 96 reports (Table 2–2) studying a total of 11,940 patients, of whom 17% were women ($n = 2,008$). No females were enrolled in 35 of the 96 studies.

Table 2–2 summarizes, by medication and number of reports, the mean and range percent participation by women. The largest trials included (N = total volunteers, percentage of females) acamprosate (3,338, 19%; Mann et al. 1995), disulfiram (605, 0%; Fuller et al. 1986; and 241, 17%; Christensen et al. 1984), lithium (457, 0%; Dorus et al. 1989), and ritanserin (423, 23%; B. A. Johnson et al. 1996). The fact that so few women are included in many trials precludes any formal analysis with respect to gender differences.

Table 2-2. Summary of gender inclusion in reports of medications for use in alcohol abuse or dependence[a]

Medication	Number of reports	Females (n)	Males (n)	Total subjects (N)	Female (%)	Female (% range)
Acamprosate	6	1,100	4,655	5,755	19.1	16.9–22.4
Bromocriptine	3	27	323	350	7.7	0–21.4
Buspirone	7	64	241	356	21.0	0–52
Calcium carbimide	4	62	247	309	20.1	0–21.1
Carbamazepine	1	11	18	29	37.9	NA
Citalopram	6	57	191	248	23.0	0–43.5
Dexfenfluramine	1	38	99	137	27.7	NA
Disulfiram	9	80	1,074	1,217	6.9	0–44.2
Enalapril	1	6	36	42	14.3	NA
Fluoxetine	12	103	351	454	22.7	0–58.3
Fluvoxamine	2	5	40	45	11.1	10–11.4
Imipramine	3	91	134	225	40.4	15.5–52.9
Lithium carbonate	8	51	995	1,046	4.9	0–12.3
Nalmefene	1	6	15	21	28.6	NA
Naltrexone	16	139	666	805	17.3	0–47.6
Nefazodone	1	9	6	15	60.0	NA
Ondansetron	1	0	71	71	0.0	NA
Ritanserin	4	109	373	482	22.6	5.6–45
Sertraline	1	6	3	9	66.7	NA
Tianeptine	1	44	86	130	33.8	NA
Tiapride	1	0	32	32	0.0	NA
Viqualine	3	0	74	74	0.0	NA
Zimelidine	4	0	88	88	0.0	NA
Total	96	2,008	9,818	11,940	17	

[a] Three reports failed to include the sex of the participants; hence, the total number of subjects exceeds the sum of females and males for buspirone and disulfiram. NA = Not applicable; only males were included in the reports.

Surprisingly, the majority of abstracts (66%) did not identify the sex of the participants. Trials with the lowest female participation have typically been conducted at Veteran's Administration hospitals (Fuller et al. 1986; Volpicelli et al. 1992) and alcohol treatment facilities (Naranjo et al. 1984, 1987, 1989, 1992) and with trials of first human exposure to drug (Sellers et al. 1994). Somewhat reassuringly, the percent inclusion of women has been steadily increasing (before 1991, 7.4 ± 12.7%; after 1991, 22.1% ± 17.1; $P < .001$). The highest female inclusion has been in trials conducted since 1991 with citalopram (44%; Naranjo et al. 1995), dexfenfluramine (27%; Romach et al. 1996), fluoxetine (49%; Cornelius et al. 1997), naltrexone (48%; Kranzler et al. 1997), sertraline (67%; Brady et al. 1995), and imipramine (53%; Nunes et al. 1993). Several of these trials were targeted to patient populations in which one would expect a higher proportion of women, such as patients with depression (Cornelius et al. 1997), anxiety, and posttraumatic stress disorder (Brady et al. 1995). In those studies that were not specifically targeted to a comorbid population, female participation was highest in those conducted at mental health treatment facilities. A noticeable trend is that, with increasing interest in and recognition of coincident mental disorders, there has been a shift in the types of medications being studied (antidepressants), the study locations, and the proportion of females participating.

When the 35 trials in which only men were enrolled were excluded, only 9 of the remaining 61 studies reported on any aspect of sex or gender on study design, recruitment, baseline characteristics, reasons for dropout, type and frequency of adverse reactions, reasons for entering treatment, retention rates, mood, alcohol consumption, or response patterns as either an assessment characteristic or an outcome predictor. In no case was this a focus of the report. Typical of the reports are incidental observations such as the findings that relatively more women than men completed the follow-up period among patients who completed the active trial period (bromocriptine; Dongier et al. 1991), and that more women were randomized by chance to the active drug condition (carbamazepine) and showed a greater decrease in drinking than the group receiving placebo (which was composed of more males) (Mueller et al. 1997). In an unpublished report, S. S. O'Malley (personal communication, October 1997) found that females had a ninefold greater frequency of side effects from naltrexone (principally nausea) than males.

Only a few trials reported on gender differences in outcome. Kranzler et al. (1995) reported that men showed a significantly greater reduction in drinks on drinking days than women in a fluoxetine trial. The study of citalopram by Naranjo et al. (1995) found that males had significantly higher scores than females on the Michigan Alcohol Screening Test (MAST) (Selzer 1971) at baseline (mean ± standard error of the mean [SEM] = 10.4 ± 0.8 versus 6.4 ± 0.9) and were heavier drinkers than females at baseline (7.1 ± 0.9 versus 5.9 ± 0.9 standard drinks per day). Citalopram (40 mg/day) was associated with a significantly greater reduction in alcohol consumption in males (44%) than in females (25.7%) (i.e., 7.1 to 4.0 ± 0.6 standard drinks per day in males and 5.9 to 4.2 ± 0.6 standard drinks per day in females). Because males had more alcohol-related problems, at least as identified by the MAST, the medication response is potentially confounded by disorder severity. The lower consumption of standard drinks in females must be interpreted cautiously. Because standard drinks are not corrected for weight or sex differences in volume of distribution, the 20% difference in consumption is very likely to reflect at least equal, and possibly greater, ethanol consumption in the females at baseline. Naranjo et al. (1995) concluded that women responded better than men to a brief psychosocial intervention but not medication, but they did not find that sex was a predictor of outcome (Naranjo et al. 1997).

One study, which was not included in our analysis because it did not include primary data, offered an interesting perspective on medication effectiveness and alcohol typology (Lesch and Walter 1996). Relying on unpublished data from the multicenter acamprosate trials performed in Austria, Switzerland, and Germany, Lesch and Walter (1996) reported that only type I and type II (and not type III or IV) alcoholic patients, as defined in the paper, responded to acamprosate. Type III alcoholic patients "consume to self-medicate" (pp. 64–65) and have periods of "minimal alcohol consumption," (p. 65), whereas type IV patients have organic brain damage. The topography of the type III alcoholic patients coincides with the pattern of drinking seen in many women, suggesting that this medication may not be effective in such women.

It is clear from this review that much work remains to be done in the development of safe and effective medications as a treatment option for alcohol use problems in women. This is a promising area of clinical research, and it is hoped that it will receive the attention and support it merits.

Summary, Conclusions, and Future Research

During the 1990s, governments, their affiliated health agencies, and the pharmaceutical industry have recognized the importance of women's health issues. In the United States, the Office of Research on Women's Health was created in the National Institutes of Health. The National Institutes of Health also mounted the Women's Health Initiative, a large study to investigate major causes of death and disability among older women, including heart disease and stroke, breast and colorectal cancer, and osteoporosis. From a public health perspective, alcohol use disorders and their treatment should also be more extensively researched in women, particularly as they interrelate with and can be risk factors in these disease states.

Women drink for different reasons than men do, and when they develop problems from alcohol use they often have concurrent psychiatric illness. Although increased work is being undertaken to address the treatment of alcohol dependence in association with these disorders, much more is needed. This needs to be supplemented by human laboratory studies to characterize the complex and different effects of ethanol in women and to explore the way alcohol serves as a reinforcer because of its mood-modulating effects. Evidence shows that once alcohol problems are present, there is a much more rapid progression of medical complications in women. This emphasizes the need for increased prevention efforts (e.g., prompt treatment of major depression, depressive symptoms, and anxiety disorders), better early recognition, and more aggressive treatment of these problems in women.

There is an urgent need for clinical treatment trials that are large enough to include sufficient male and female subjects for independent analysis of effects on women. Clinical trial reports should routinely report sex distribution in the abstracts of their trials, and specific mention of a gender effect should be made for every dependent variable. Treatment inclusion and outcome measures need to incorporate what is known about levels of hazardous drinking in women, risk, and differences in alcohol disposition. Further research is needed to determine which treatment modalities are specifically effective for women and for men.

References

Abrams D, Niaura RS: Social learning theory, in Psychological Theories of Drinking and Alcoholism. Edited by Blane HT, Leonard KE. New York, Guilford, 1987, pp 131–178

Acker C: Performance of female alcoholics on neuropsychological testing. Alcohol Alcohol 20(4):379–386, 1985

American Psychiatric Association: Diagnostic and Statistical Manual of Mental Disorders, 3rd Edition, Revised. Washington, DC, American Psychiatric Association, 1987

American Psychiatric Association: Diagnostic and Statistical Manual of Mental Disorders, 4th Edition. Washington, DC, American Psychiatric Association, 1994

Ammon E, Schäfer C, Hofmann U, et al: Disposition and first-pass metabolism of ethanol in humans: is it gastric or hepatic and does it depend on gender? Clin Pharmacol Ther 59(5):503–513, 1996

Ballinger S: Stress as a factor in lowered estrogen levels in the early postmenopause. Ann N Y Acad Sci 592:95–113, 1991

Beck AT, Steer RA, McElroy MG: Self-reported precedence of depression in alcoholism. Drug Alcohol Depend 10:185–190, 1982

Beck SG, Clarke WP, Goldfarb J: Chronic estrogen effects on 5-hydroxy-tryptamine-mediated responses in hippocampal pyramidal cells of female rats. Neurosci Lett 106:181–187, 1989

Becker U: The influence of ethanol and liver disease on sex hormones and hepatic estrogen receptors in women. Dan Med Bull 4:447–457, 1993

Belfer ML, Shader RI: Premenstrual factors as determinants of alcoholism in women, in Alcohol Problems in Women and Children. Edited by Greenblatt M, Schuckit MA. New York, Grune & Stratton, 1976, pp 97–102

Bitran D, Purdy RH, Kellogg CK: Anxiolytic effect of progesterone is associated with increases in cortical allopregnanolone and $GABA_A$ receptor function. Pharmacol Biochem Behav 45:423–428, 1993

Brady KT, Sonne SC, Roberts JM: Sertraline treatment of comorbid posttraumatic stress disorder and alcohol dependence. J Clin Psychiatry 56(11):502–505, 1995

Brick J, Nathan PE, Westrick E, et al: The effect of menstrual cycle on blood alcohol levels and behavior. J Stud Alcohol 47:472–477, 1986

Brot MD, Koob FG, Britton KT: Anxiolytic effects of steroid hormones during the estrous cycle: interactions with alcohol, in Recent Developments in Alcoholism, Vol 12. Edited by Galanter M. New York, Plenum, 1995, pp 243–259

Brown SA: Reinforcement expectancies and alcoholism treatment outcome. Addict Behav 10:191–195, 1985

Burns M, Moskowitz H: Gender-related differences in impairment of performance by alcohol, in Currents in Alcoholism, Vol 3. Biological, Biochemical and Clinical Studies. Edited by Seixas F. New York, Grune & Stratton, 1978, pp 479–492

Cappell H, Greeley J: Alcohol and tension reduction: an update on research and theory, in Psychological Theories of Drinking and Alcoholism. Edited by Blane HT, Leonard KE. New York, Guilford, 1987, pp 15–54

Carey MP, Billing AE, Fry JP: Fluctuations in responses to diazepam during the oestrous cycle in the mouse. Pharmacol Biochem Behav 41:719–725, 1992

Chan AWK: Recent developments in detection and biological indicators of alcoholism. Drugs and Society 8:31–67, 1993

Charette L, Tate DL, Wilson A: Alcohol consumption and menstrual distress in women at higher and lower risk for alcoholism. Alcohol Clin Exp Res 14:152–157, 1990

Christensen JK, Rønsted P, Vaag UH: Side effects after disulfiram: comparison of disulfiram and placebo in a double-blind multicentre study. Acta Psychiatr Scand 69:265–273, 1984

Ciraulo DA, Sarid-Segal O, Knapp C, et al: Liability to alprazolam abuse in daughters of alcoholics. Am J Psychiatry 153(7):956–958, 1996

Corcoran KJ, Parker PS: Alcohol expectancy questionnaire tension reduction as a predictor of alcohol consumption in a stressful situation. Addict Behav 16:129–137, 1991

Cornelius JR, Salloum IM, Ehler JG, et al: Fluoxetine in depressed alcoholics: a double-blind, placebo-controlled trial. Arch Gen Psychiatry 54:700–705, 1997

Cox BJ, Swinson RP, Shulman ID, et al: Gender effects and alcohol use in panic disorder with agoraphobia. Behav Res Ther 31:413–416, 1993

Davidson D, Camara P, Swift R: Behavioral effects and pharmacokinetics of low-dose intravenous alcohol in humans. Alcohol Clin Exp Res 21(7):1294–1299, 1997

Deal SR, Gavaler JS: Are women more susceptible than men to alcohol-induced cirrhosis? Alcohol Health Res World 18:189–191, 1994

de Boer MC, Schippers GM, Van Der Staak CPF: Alcohol and social anxiety in women and men: pharmacological and expectancy effects. Addict Behav 18:117–126, 1993

de Wit H, Chutuape MA: Increased ethanol choice in social drinkers following ethanol preload. Behav Pharmacol 4:29–36, 1993

Dongier M, Vachon L, Schwartz G: Bromocriptine in the treatment of alcohol dependence. Alcohol Clin Exp Res 15(6):970–979, 1991

Dorgan JF, Reichman ME, Judd JT, et al: The relation of reported alcohol ingestion to plasma levels of estrogens and androgens in premenopausal women (Maryland, United States). Cancer Causes and Control 5:53–60, 1994

Dorus W, Ostrow DG, Anton R, et al: Lithium treatment of depressed and nondepressed alcoholics. JAMA 262(12):1646–1652, 1989

Drake AI, Hannay HJ, Gam J: Effects of chronic alcoholism on hemispheric functioning: an examination of gender differences for cognitive and dichotic listening tasks. J Clin Exp Neuropsychol 12(5):781–797, 1990

Felson DT, Zhang Y, Hannan MT, et al: Alcohol intake and bone mineral density in elderly men and women: the Framingham study. Am J Epidemiol 142(5):485–492, 1995

Frezza MR, Di Padova C, Pozzato G, et al: High blood and alcohol levels in women: the role of decreased alcohol dehydrogenase activity and first-pass metabolism. N Engl J Med 322(2):95–99, 1990

Fuller RK, Branchey L, Brightwell DR, et al: Disulfiram treatment of alcoholism: a Veterans Administration Cooperative Study. JAMA 256(11):1449–1455, 1986

Gavaler JS, Van Thiel DH: The association between moderate alcoholic beverage consumption and serum estradiol and testosterone levels in normal postmenopausal women: relationship to the literature. Alcohol Clin Exp Res 16:87–92, 1992

George DT, Benkelfat C, Rawlings RR, et al: Behavioral and neuroendocrine responses to m-chlorophenylpiperazine in subtypes of alcoholics and in healthy comparison subjects. Am J Psychiatry 154(1):81–87, 1997

Ginsburg ES, Walsh BW, Gao X, et al: The effects of acute ethanol ingestion on estrogen levels in post-menopausal women using transdermal estradiol. J Soc Gynecol Invest 2:26–29, 1995

Ginsburg ES, Mello NK, Mendelson JH, et al: Effects of alcohol ingestion on estrogens in postmenopausal women. JAMA 276(21):1747–1751, 1996

Goldman M, Brown S, Christiansen B: Expectancy theory: thinking about drinking, in Psychological Theories of Drinking and Alcoholism. Edited by Blane HT, Leonard KE. New York, Guilford, 1987, pp 181–226

Gorman DM: Distinguishing primary and secondary disorders in studies of alcohol dependence and depression. Drug Alcohol Rev 11:23–29, 1992

Gotlieb IH, Lewinsohn PM, Seeley JR: Symptoms as a diagnosis of depression: differences in psychosocial functioning. J Consult Clin Psychol 63:90–100, 1995

Grant BF, Harford TC: Comorbidity between DSM-IV alcohol use disorders and major depression: results of a national survey. Drug Alcohol Depend 39:197–206, 1995

Gustafson R: Is the strength and the desirability of alcohol related expectancies positively related? A test with an adult Swedish sample. Drug Alcohol Depend 28:145–150, 1991

Harris RZ, Benet LZ, Schwartz JB: Gender effects in pharmacokinetics and pharmacodynamics. Drugs 50(2):222–239, 1995

Hatsukami D, Pickens RW: Post-treatment depression in an alcohol and drug abuse population. Am J Psychiatry 139:1563–1566, 1982

Helzer JE, Pryzbeck TR: The co-occurrence of alcoholism with other psychiatric disorders in the general population and its impact on treatment. J Stud Alcohol 49:219–224, 1988

Hilakivi-Clarke L: Role of estradiol in alcohol intake and alcohol related behaviors. J Stud Alcohol 57:162–170, 1996

Hugues JN, Coste T, Perret G, et al: Hypothalamo-pituitary ovarian function in 31 women with chronic alcoholism. Clin Endocrinol 12(6):543—551, 1980

Jaffe JH, Ciraulo DA: Alcoholism and depression, in Psychopathology and Addictive Disorders. Edited by Meyer RE. New York, Guilford, 1986, pp 293–320

Johnson BA, Jasinski DR, Galloway GP, et al: Ritanserin in the treatment of alcohol dependence—a multi-center clinical trial. Psychopharmacology 128:206–215, 1996

Johnson LD, O'Malley PM, Backman JG: National Survey Results on Drug Use From the Monitoring the Future Study, 1975–1993, Vol II: College Students and Young Adults. NIH Publication No 94-3810. Washington, DC, U.S. Government Printing Office, 1994

Jones BM, Jones MK: Alcohol effects in women during the menstrual cycle. Ann N Y Acad Sci 273:576–587, 1976

Kendler KS, Heath AC, Neale MC, et al: Alcoholism and major depression in women: a twin study of the causes of comorbidity. Arch Gen Psychiatry 50(9):690–698, 1993

Kessler RC, McGonagle KA, Zhao S, et al: Lifetime and 12 month prevalence of DSM-III-R psychiatric disorders in the United States: results from the National Comorbidity Survey. Arch Gen Psychiatry 51(1):8–19, 1994

Kranzler HR, del Boca F, Rounsaville B: Psychopathology as a predictor of outcome three years after alcoholism treatment (abstract). Alcohol Clin Exp Res 16(2):363, 1992

Kranzler HR, Burleson JA, Korner P, et al: Placebo-controlled trial of fluoxetine as an adjunct to relapse prevention in alcoholics. Am J Psychiatry 152(3):391–397, 1995

Kranzler HR, Tennen H, Penta C, et al: Targeted naltrexone treatment of early problem drinkers. Addict Behav 22(3):431–436, 1997

Kushner MG, Sher KJ: Comorbidity of alcohol and anxiety disorders among college students: effects of gender and family history of alcoholism. Addict Behav 18:543–552, 1993

Kushner MG, Sher KJ, Wood DW, et al: Anxiety and drinking behavior: moderating effects of tension-reduction alcohol outcome expectancies. Alcohol Clin Exp Res 18:852–860, 1994

Lammers S, Mainzer D, Breteler HM: Do alcohol pharmacokinetics in women vary due to the menstrual cycle? Addiction 90:23–30, 1995

Leigh BC: In search of the seven dwarves: issues of measurement and meaning in alcohol expectancy research. Psychol Bull 105:361–373, 1989

Lesch OM, Walter H: Subtypes of alcoholism and their role in therapy. Alcohol Alcohol 31 (suppl 1):63–67, 1996

Lex BW, Lukas SE, Greenwald NE, et al: Alcohol-induced changes in body sway in women at risk for alcoholism: a pilot study. J Stud Alcohol 49(4):346–356, 1988

Liebenluft E, Fiero PL, Bartko JJ, et al: Depressive symptoms and the self-reported use of alcohol, caffeine and carbohydrates in normal volunteers and four groups of psychiatric outpatients. Am J Psychiatry 150:294–301, 1993

Lieber CS: Gender differences in alcohol metabolism and susceptibility, in Gender and Alcohol: Individual and Social Perspectives. Edited by Wilsnack RW, Wilsnack SC. New Brunswick, NJ, Alcohol Research Documentation, 1997, pp 77–89

Litt MD, Cooney NL, Kadden RM, et al: Reactivity to alcohol cues induced moods in alcoholics. Addict Behav 15:137–146, 1990

Malcolm R, Anton RF, Randall CL, et al: A placebo-controlled trial of buspirone in anxious inpatient alcoholics. Alcohol Clin Exp Res 16:1007–1013, 1992

Mann K, Batra A, Gunthner A, et al: Do women develop alcoholic brain damage more readily than men? Alcohol Clin Exp Res 16(6):1052–1056, 1992

Mann K, Chabac S, Lehert P, et al: Acamprosate improves treatment outcome in alcoholics: a pooled analysis of 11 randomized placebo controlled trials in 3338 patients. Poster presented at the Annual Conference of the American College of Neuropsychopharmacology, San Juan, Puerto Rico, December 1995

Marlatt GA, Gordon JR: Determinants of relapse: implications for the maintenance of behavior change, in Behavioral Medicine: Changing Health Lifestyles. Edited by Davidson PO, Davidson SM. New York, Brunner/Mazel, 1985, pp 410–452

Mason BJ, Ritro EC, Morgan RO, et al: A double-blind, placebo-controlled pilot study to evaluate the efficacy and safety of oral nalmefine HCl for alcohol dependence. Alcohol Clin Exp Res 18:1162–1167, 1994

Mason BJ, Kocsis JH, Ritvo EC, et al: A double-blind, placebo-controlled trial of desipramine for primary alcohol dependence stratified on the presence or absence of major depression. JAMA 275(10):761–767, 1996

Mayfield DG: Alcohol and affect: experimental studies, in Alcoholism and Affective Disorders. Edited by Goodwin DW, Erickson CK. New York, Spectrum, 1979, pp 288–290

McAuley JW, Reynolds IJ, Kroboth FJ, et al: Orally administered progesterone enhances sensitivity to triazolam in post-menopausal women. J Clin Psychopharmacol 15:3–11, 1995

McGrath PJ, Nunes EV, Stewart JW, et al: Imipramine treatment of alcoholics with primary depression: a placebo controlled clinical trial. Arch Gen Psychiatry 53(3):232–240, 1996

Mello NK: Some behavior and biological aspects of alcohol problems in women, in Alcohol and Drug Problems in Women, Vol 5. Edited by Kalant H. New York, Plenum, 1980, pp 263–298

Mendelson JH, Lukas SE, Mellow NK, et al: Acute alcohol effects on plasma estradiol levels in women. Psychopharmacology 94:464–467, 1988

Merikangas KR, Gelernter CS: Comorbidity for alcoholism and depression. Psychiatry Clin North Am 13(4):613–632, 1990

Midanik LT, Clark WB: The demographic distribution of US drinking patterns in 1990: description and trends from 1984. Am J Public Health 84:1218–1222, 1994

Mills KC, Bisgrove EZ: Body sway and divided attention performance under the influence of alcohol: dose-response differences between males and females. Alcohol Clin Exp Res 7:393–397, 1983

Moskovic S: Effect of chronic alcohol intoxication on ovarian dysfunction. Srp Arh Celok Lek 103:751–758, 1975

Mueller TI, Stout RL, Rudden S, et al: A double-blind, placebo-controlled pilot study of carbamazepine for the treatment of alcohol dependence. Alcohol Clin Exp Res 21(1):86–92, 1997

Naranjo CA, Sellers EM, Roach CA, et al: Zimelidine-induced variations in alcohol intake by non-depressed heavy drinkers. Clin Pharmacol Ther 35:374–381, 1984

Naranjo CA, Sellers EM, Sullivan JT, et al: The serotonin uptake inhibitor citalopram attenuates ethanol intake. Clin Pharmacol Ther 41(3):266–274, 1987

Naranjo CA, Sullivan JT, Kadlec KE, et al: Differential effects of viqualine on alcohol intake and other consummatory behaviors. Clin Pharmacol Ther 46(3):301–309, 1989

Naranjo CA, Kadlec KE, Sanhueza P, et al: Fluoxetine differentially alters alcohol intake and other consummatory behaviors in problem drinkers. Clin Pharmacol Ther 47(4):490–498, 1990

Naranjo CA, Poulos CV, Bremner KE, et al: Citalopram decreases desirability, liking and consumption of alcohol in alcohol dependent drinkers. Clin Pharmacol Ther 51:729–739, 1992

Naranjo CA, Bremner KE, Lanctôt KL: Effects of citalopram and a brief psychosocial intervention on alcohol intake, dependence and problems. Addiction 90:87–99, 1995

Naranjo CA, Bremner KE, Bazoon M, et al: Using fuzzy logic to predict response to citalopram in alcohol dependence. Clin Pharmacol Ther 62(2):209–224, 1997

Neve RJM, Drop MJ, Lemmens PH, et al: Gender differences in drinking behaviour in the Netherlands: convergence or stability. Addiction 91(3):357–373, 1996

Niaura RS, Nathan PE, Frankenstein W, et al: Gender differences in acute psychomotor, cognitive, and pharmacokinetic response to alcohol. Addict Behav 12:345–356, 1987

Nunes EV, McGrath PJ, Quitkin FM, et al: Imipramine treatment of alcoholism with comorbid depression. Am J Psychiatry 150(5):963–965, 1993

O'Malley SS, Jaffe A, Chang G, et al: Naltrexone and coping skills therapy for alcohol dependence: a controlled study. Arch Gen Psychiatry 49:881–887, 1992

Penick EC, Powell BJ, Liskow BI, et al: The stability of co-existing psychiatric syndromes in alcoholic men after one year. J Stud Alcohol 49:395–405, 1988

Perkins HW: Gender patterns in consequences of collegiate alcohol abuse: a 10-year study of trends in an undergraduate population. J Stud Alcohol 53:458–462, 1992

Reiger DA, Farmer ME, Rae DS, et al: Comorbidity of mental disorders with alcohol and other drug abuse. JAMA 264:2511–2518, 1990

Romach MK, Somer G, Kaplan HL, et al: The three faces of depression and alcohol dependence. Abstracts of Science Day, Addiction Research Foundation, Toronto, Ontario, April 1995

Romach MK, Sellers EM, Kaplan HL, et al: Efficacy of dexfenfluramine (DEX) in the treatment of alcohol dependence. Alcohol Clin Exp Res 20(2):90A, 1996

Ross HE: DSM-III-R alcohol abuse and dependence and psychiatric comorbidity in Ontario: results from the Mental Health Supplement to the Ontario Health Survey. Drug Alcohol Depend 39:111–128, 1995

Ross H, Glaser FB, Stiasny S: Sex differences in the prevalence of psychiatric disorders in patients with alcohol and drug problems. Br J Addict 83(10):1179–1192, 1988a

Ross HE, Glaser FB, Germanson T: The prevalence of psychiatric disorders in patients with alcohol and other drug problems. Arch Gen Psychiatry 45:1023–1031, 1988b

Rounsaville BJ, Dolinsky Z, Babor TF, et al: Psychopathology as a predictor of treatment outcome in alcoholics. Arch Gen Psychiatry 44:505–513, 1987

Sass H, Soyka M, Mann K, et al: Relapse prevention by acamprosate: results from a placebo-controlled study on alcohol dependence. Arch Gen Psychiatry 53:673–680, 1996

Schober R, Annis HM: Barriers to help-seeking for change in drinking: a gender-focused review of the literature. Addict Behav 21(1):81–92, 1996

Schuckit MA: Genetic and clinical implications of alcoholism and affective disorder. Am J Psychiatry 143:140–147, 1986

Schutte KK, Moos RH, Brennan PL: Depression and drinking behaviour among women and men: a three-wave longitudinal study of older adults. J Consult Clin Psychol 63:810–822, 1995

Sellers EM, Higgins GA, Tomkins DM, et al: Opportunities for treatment of psychoactive substance use disorders with serotonergic medications. J Clin Psychiatry 52 (suppl):49–54, 1991

Sellers EM, Toneatto T, Romach MK, et al: Clinical efficacy of the 5-HT3 antagonist ondansetron in alcohol abuse and dependence. Alcohol Clin Exp Res 18(4):879–885, 1994

Selzer ML: The Michigan Alcohol Screening Test: the quest for a new diagnostic instrument. Am J Psychiatry 127:1653–1658, 1971

Sher KJ: Subjective effects of alcohol: the influence of setting and individual differences in alcohol expectancies. J Stud Alcohol 46:137–146, 1985

Steele CM, Josephs RA: Drinking your troubles away, II: an attention allocation model of alcohol's effect on psychological stress. J Abnorm Psychol 97:196–205, 1988

Sutker PB, Allain AN, Brantley PS, et al: Acute alcohol intoxication, negative affect, and autonomic arousal in women and men. Addict Behav 7:17–25, 1982

Sutker PB, Libet JM, Allain AN, et al: Alcohol use, negative mood states and menstrual cycle phases. Alcohol Clin Exp Res 7:327–331, 1983

Taberner PV: Sex differences in the effects of low doses of ethanol on human reaction time. Psychopharmacology 70:283–286, 1980

Thom B: Sex differences in help-seeking for alcohol problems, I: the barriers to help-seeking. Br J Addict 81:777–788, 1986

Thomasson HR: Gender differences in alcohol metabolism: physiological responses to ethanol, in Recent Developments in Alcoholism, Vol 12: Women and Alcoholism. Edited by Galanter M. New York, Plenum, 1995, pp 163–179

Thomasson HR, Beard JD, Li T-K: Gender differences in ethanol metabolism. Alcohol Clin Exp Res 18:921, 1994

Tollefson GD, Montague-Clouse J, Tollefson SL: Treatment of comorbid generalized anxiety in a recently detoxified alcohol population with a selective serotonergic drug (buspirone). J Clin Psychopharmacol 12:19–26, 1992

Turnbull JE, Gomberg ES: Impact of depressive symptomatology on alcohol problems in women. Alcohol Clin Exp Res 12(3):374–381, 1988

Turnbull JE, Gomberg ES: The structure of depression in alcoholic women. J Stud Alcohol 51(2):148–155, 1990

Urbano-Márquez A, Estruch R, Fernández-Solá J, et al: The greater risk of alcoholic cardiomyopathy and myopathy in women compared with men. JAMA 274(2):149–155, 1995

Van Thiel DH, Gavaler JS, Rosenblum E, et al: Ethanol, its metabolism and hepatotoxicity as well as its gonadal effects: effects of sex. Pharmacol Ther 41:27–48, 1989

Volk RJ, Steinbauer JR, Cantor SB: Patient factors influencing variation in the use of preventive interventions for alcohol abuse by primary care physicians. J Stud Alcohol 57:203–209, 1996

Volpicelli JR, Alterman AI, Hayashida M, et al: Naltrexone in the treatment of alcohol dependence. Arch Gen Psychiatry 49:876–880, 1992

von Korff M, Ormel J, Katon W, et al: Disability and depression among high utilizers of health care. Arch Gen Psychiatry 49:91–100, 1992

Wait JS, Welch RB, Thurgate JK, et al: Drinking history and sex of subject in the effects of alcohol on perception and perceptual-motor coordination. Int J Addict 17:445–462, 1982

Wheatley D: Depression and the menopause. Br J Psychiatry 158:431–432, 1991

Wilsnack SC, Wilsnack RW, Hiller-Sturmhöfel S: How women drink: epidemiology of women's drinking and problem drinking. Alcohol Health Res World 18(3):173–181, 1994

Wilson GT: Alcohol and anxiety. Behav Ther Res 26:369–381, 1988

Yanofsky L, Wilson GT, Adler JL, et al: The effect of alcohol on self-evaluation and perception of negative interpersonal feedback. J Stud Alcohol 47(1):26–35, 1986

Young RM, Longmore BE: Alcohol related beliefs and treatment success. Paper presented at the International Symposium of Alcohol and the Brain, Brisbane, Australia, August 1987

Chapter 3

Opiate Dependence and Current Treatments

Susan M. Stine, M.D., Ph.D.

Opiate Dependence

Opiate dependence has been a continuous public health problem throughout this century, and now, on the eve of the next, it shows no sign of decline—rather, a new epidemic is in progress. Because opioids are tightly regulated, especially in the United States, demand by addicted persons results in crime, disease, poverty, and loss of personal and social productivity. Prostitution is closely linked with drug abuse in general and opioid use in particular and contributes to the spread of HIV infection, as well as other sexually transmitted and infectious diseases. High overall death rates are associated with opioid abuse. Opioids typically consume the individual's attention, resources, and energy, focusing these exclusively on obtaining the next dose at any cost. The consequent pervasive personal deterioration leads to the need for long-term treatments and intense psychosocial interventions.

Current Epidemiological Trends

During the last 5 years, a substantial new epidemic of heroin abuse has been developing in the United States and has been spreading to middle-class users, who formerly were more likely to abuse only cocaine. *Pulse Check,* a publication by the Office of National Drug Control Policy, reported in December 1994 four key trends in heroin use: 1) more teenagers and young adults are using heroin; 2) more middle- and upper-middle class people are using heroin; 3) the heroin being used is purer; and 4) the proportion of people inhaling or smoking heroin, as well as the number of people seeking treatment, continues to increase. The National Drug Control Strategy reports that the strongest sign of an epidemic is the incidence of a large number of new users (new initiates), and this new influx of heroin users defines such an epidemic. Because they have had less exposure and fewer chronic health problems (at least with respect to infectious disease) and legal adverse consequences, new users are more likely to recruit other new users.

Many drug abusers mistakenly believe that inhaling heroin, rather than injecting it, reduces the risks of addiction or overdose. In some areas, "shabanging"—picking up cooked heroin with a syringe and squirting it up the nose—has increased in popularity. Previously commonly known as "smack" or "horse" for years, the new, pure heroin is more life-threatening, a fact reflected in the new street terminology: "DOA," "Body Bag," "Instant Death," and "Silence of the Lamb." The implied danger seems to actually increase the drug's allure (AT Forum 1997).

The expanding market for heroin fortunately coincides with the availability of a variety of new treatments. These include developments in the treatment of acute withdrawal and chronic dependence with antagonist and agonist pharmacotherapy, new ways to optimize the delivery of methadone maintenance, and newly available breakthrough pharmacotherapies.

Diagnosis

The previous DSM-III-R (American Psychiatric Association 1987) categories of substance use disorders and substance-induced disorders are now grouped under "Substance-Related Disorders" in DSM-IV (American Psychiatric Association 1994). The concept of substance dependence has been clarified, and where substance abuse was a residual category without a clear framework, it is now conceptualized as a maladaptive pattern of substance use that leads to adverse consequences in the absence of substance dependence. A table of substance-induced disorders has also been expanded in DSM-IV and incorporates much interesting clinical material.

Opiate use presents clinically as two separate classes of signs and symptoms: those of acute use and those of chronic use. Although mild opioid intoxication and opioid withdrawal are not usually life threatening, severe intoxication or overdose is a medical emergency that requires immediate attention. Of primary concern in the management of overdose are sedation and respiratory depression. Miosis ("pinpoint pupils") is an important pharmacological effect that can be used as a sign to identify possible opioid intoxication.

The triad of coma, pinpoint pupils, and depressed respiration strongly suggests opioid poisoning. Because this often occurs in combination with other drugs, pharmacological therapy for opiate dependence, as well as screening for the presence of other drugs and metabolites, should be instituted immediately. The finding of needle marks suggestive of addiction further supports the diagnosis. Examination of the urine and gastric contents for drugs may aid in diagnosis, but the results usually become available too late to influence treatment.

Two prominent physiological features of chronic opiate use have been described: tolerance, characterized by a diminishing drug effect after repeated administration; and dependence, revealed by a withdrawal syndrome after abrupt discontinuation of opiate exposure. Opioids are also psychologically addicting in that their effects are acutely reinforcing and produce escalating drug-seeking behavior with repeated exposure.

Withdrawal from opioids results in a specific constellation of symptoms in addition to some relatively nonspecific symptoms. Clinical phenomena associated with opioid withdrawal generally consist of symptoms related to neurophysiological rebound in the organ systems on which opioids have their primary actions. The severity of opioid withdrawal varies with the dose and duration of drug use. The time to onset of opioid withdrawal symptoms depends on the half-life of the drug being used. For example, withdrawal may begin 4–6 hours after the last use of heroin but up to 36 hours after the last use of methadone (Gold et al. 1980). Early findings may include abnormalities in vital signs, including tachycardia and hypertension. Pupillary dilation can be marked. Central nervous system (CNS) symptoms include restlessness, irritability, and insomnia. Opioid craving also occurs in proportion to the severity of physiological withdrawal symptoms. Patients frequently note yawning and sneezing, gastrointestinal symptoms (which initially may be simply anorexia but can progress to include nausea, vomiting, and diarrhea), and a variety of cutaneous and mucocutaneous symptoms (including lacrimation, rhinorrhea, and piloerection, also known as "gooseflesh"). This combination of symptomatology and intense craving frequently leads to relapse to drug use. Although some opioid withdrawal symptoms overlap with withdrawal from sedative-hypnotics, opioid withdrawal generally is considered less likely to produce severe morbidity or mortality.

Foundations for Current Treatment

Advances in the behavioral psychology of addiction and in basic neurobiology have formed the foundation of the new treatments for opiate dependence. Animal models allow control over a variety of factors, including genetic background; environmental influences; and types and lengths of prior experiences, such as drug exposure (Gallup and Suarez 1985). The behavioral techniques used to assess the acute and chronic effects of opioid exposure in animals include assessments of unconditioned effects of opioids as well as measures acquired from procedures involving classical and operant conditioning principles, such as place conditioning, self-administration, and drug discrimination.

Animal models have contributed to the development of pharmacological treatment agents as well as to the relapse prevention psychotherapy approach to treating drug and alcohol abuse. Cues in the environment—for example, the sight of the place where the drug is bought—that were reliably associated with drug procurement or drug use can elicit drug-opposing or drug withdrawal-like effects. Relapse prevention helps the addicted person to recognize and deal with these effects as one aspect of maintaining drug abstinence.

The discovery of opioid receptors raised the possibility that dependence and tolerance could be explained in terms of changes in these receptors. There are three major classes of opioid receptors in the CNS, designated μ, δ, and κ, as well as subtypes within each class. Members of each class of opioid receptor have been cloned from human cyclic DNA and their predicted amino acid sequences obtained. Their amino acid sequences are approximately 65% identical, and they have little sequence similarity to other G protein–coupled receptors except those for somatostatin (Reisine and Bell 1993). Regions that differ in amino acid sequence are the amino and carboxy termini and the second and third extracellular loops. The extracellular regions contain the unique ligand-binding domains of each receptor.

There have been numerous claims over the years, based on classical pharmacological binding studies and pharmacological effects on intact animals, that multiple subtypes for the μ, δ, and κ receptors exist in the brain. However, the molecular basis of some of these variants that has been described by binding, pharmacology, and behavior studies remains uncertain, because molecular cloning studies have so far failed to confirm them, notably $\mu 1$ and $\mu 2$ (Reisine and Pasternak 1996). They all appear to be coupled to the guanidine nucleotide, which is involved in the subcellular mechanisms of addiction.

Of the endogenous opioid peptides, β-endorphin has the greatest affinity for μ receptors, enkephalins for δ receptors, and dynorphin for κ receptors. With respect to psychological addiction to opiates, μ and δ receptors are primarily implicated in mediating the reinforcing actions of opiates and κ receptors in mediating their aversive actions (Reisine and Pasternak 1996). However, opioids that are relatively selective at standard doses will interact with additional receptor classes when given at sufficiently high doses. This is especially true as doses are escalated to overcome tolerance. Some drugs, particularly mixed agonist-antagonist agents, interact with more than one receptor class at usual clinical doses, and they may act as an agonist at one receptor and an antagonist at another.

Numerous receptor binding studies have been carried out to investigate the changes induced by chronic opioid exposure, but most have failed to detect changes in opiate binding (Nestler et al. 1993). In contrast to the difficulty in establishing consistent effects of chronic opioid exposure on receptors, studies of the chronic effects of opiates on postreceptor signal transduction pathways have been more fruitful (Nestler et al. 1993). Opioids regulate adenyl cyclase, Ca^{2+} channels, and phosphatidylinositol turnover, suggesting that they may also produce changes in cyclic adenosine monophosphate (cAMP)-dependent and calcium-dependent protein phosphorylation in specific target neurons. Chronic exposure to opioids has been shown to produce long-term changes in levels of specific G protein subunits and in the individual proteins that make up the cAMP system, but a definitive demonstration of opioid receptor phosphorylation has yet to appear. The subject of subcellular mechanisms of addiction has been extensively reviewed by Nestler (1997).

Many regions of the CNS are opioid responsive, but three well-characterized neuroanatomical systems are most important: 1) the mesolimbic dopamine system, 2) pathways originating from and impinging upon the locus ceruleus (LC), and 3) the dorsal root ganglion-spinal cord. The first two systems are the most relevant to addictive actions and have provided particularly useful model systems in which to study the mechanisms underlying the acute and chronic actions of opiates on the nervous system.

Increasing evidence indicates that the mesolimbic dopamine system—consisting of dopaminergic neurons in the ventral tegmental area and their projection regions, most notably the nucleus accumbens—plays an important role in mediating the reinforcing actions of opiates on brain function. Animals will self-administer opiates directly into the ventral tegmental area and nucleus accumbens and will develop conditioned place preference after such local drug administration (Wise 1990).

The LC, located on the floor of the fourth ventricle in the anterior pons, is the major noradrenergic nucleus in the brain and has widespread projections to both the brain and the spinal cord. An important role for the LC in opiate physical dependence and withdrawal has been established at both the behavioral and the electrophysiological level. During abstinent states, overactivation of LC neurons and increased release of norepinephrine is both necessary and sufficient for producing many of the behavioral signs of withdrawal (Aghajanian 1978; see Nestler et al. 1993 for a review and model). Acute opioid administration decreases norepinephrine release, whereas chronically, LC neurons develop tolerance to acute inhibitory actions of opiates as neuronal activity recovers toward preexposure levels (Aghajanian 1978). Abrupt cessation of opiate treatment, for example, via administration of an opioid receptor antagonist, causes a marked increase in neuronal firing rates above preexposure levels both in vivo and in isolated slice preparations (Aghajanian 1978). Overactivation of LC neurons during withdrawal arises from both extrinsic and intrinsic sources. The extrinsic source involves a hyperactive excitatory glutaminergic input to the LC. The intrinsic source involves intracellular adaptations in signal transduction pathways coupled to opioid receptors in the LC neurons.

The discovery of the importance of noradrenergic mechanisms as described above led to clinical therapies such as clonidine administration (described below), which is designed to alter the course of opioid withdrawal by decreasing this LC hyperactivity (by acting on presynaptic receptors) (Gold et al. 1980).

In addition to dopaminergic and noradrenergic mechanisms, excitatory amino acids are also a recent focus of interest. For example, blockade of glutamate actions by noncompetitive and competitive NMDA (N-methyl-D-aspartate) antagonists blocks morphine tolerance (Trujillo and Akil 1991). Because these NMDA antagonists have no effect on the potency of morphine in naive animals, their effect cannot be attributed to a simple potentiation of opioid actions. Blockade of the glycine regulatory site on NMDA receptors also has the ability to block tolerance. Inhibition of nitric oxide synthase blocks morphine tolerance and reverses tolerance in morphine-tolerant animals, despite continued opioid administration. Although the NMDA antagonists and nitric oxide synthase inhibitors are effective against tolerance to morphine and other μ agonists, they have little effect against tolerance to the κ agonists. Dependence seems to be closely related to tolerance, because the same treatments that block tolerance to morphine also often block dependence. Co-administration of the α_2-adrenergic antagonist yohimbine, however, has been reported to prevent naloxone-precipitated withdrawal (dependence) in animals without diminishing the analgesic effect (tolerance) (Taylor et al. 1991). It may therefore be possible to differentially affect these phenomena.

Traditional Treatments

Pharmacotherapy

Acute Treatments for Opiate Intoxication, Overdose, and Withdrawal

Naloxone hydrochloride, a pure opioid antagonist, can effectively reverse the CNS effects of opioid intoxication and overdose. An initial intravenous dose of 0.4–0.8 mg dramatically (in approximately 2 minutes) reverses neurological and cardiorespiratory depression, but care should be taken to avoid precipitating withdrawal in dependent patients who may be extremely sensitive to antagonists. The safest approach is to dilute the standard naloxone dose (0.4 mg) and slowly administer it intravenously, monitoring arousal and respiratory function. With care, it usually is possible to reverse respiratory depression without precipitating a major withdrawal syndrome. If no response is seen with the first dose, additional doses can be given. Patients should be observed for rebound increases in sympathetic nervous system activity, which may result in cardiac arrhythmia and pulmonary edema (Reisine and Pasternak 1996). Pulmonary edema sometimes associated with opioid overdose may be countered by positive-pressure respiration. Tonic-clonic seizures, occasionally seen as part of the toxic syndrome with meperidine and propoxyphene, are ameliorated by treatment with naloxone. Overdose with more potent (e.g., fentanyl) or longer acting opioids (methadone) may require higher doses of naloxone given over longer periods of time, thus necessitating the use of ongoing naloxone infusion.

Abstinence from opioids after chronic exposure typically produces withdrawal, the onset and duration of which varies with the drug used. In patients hospitalized for medical illnesses, the severity of the underlying clinical conditions can also alter the selection of withdrawal therapy (O'Connor et al. 1994). The decision of whether to perform opioid detoxification on an outpatient or an inpatient basis depends on the presence of comorbid medical and psychiatric problems, the availability of social support (e.g., family members to provide monitoring and transportation) and the presence of polydrug abuse. The available methods of detoxification may also affect this decision; for example, methadone detoxification is legally restricted by federal legislation to inpatient settings or specialized licensed outpatient drug treatment programs.

A variety of pharmacological therapies have been developed to assist patients through a safer, more comfortable opioid withdrawal. These therapies involve the use of opioid agonists (e.g., methadone), α_2-adrenergic agonists such as clonidine, the opioid antagonist naltrexone in combination with clonidine, and a mixed opioid agonist-antagonist, buprenorphine.

The simplest approach to detoxification is to substitute a prescribed opioid for the heroin (or opioid) on which the addicted individual is dependent and then gradually lower the dose of the prescribed opioid. The prescribed agent commonly is methadone, but l-α-acetylmethadol (LAAM) can also be used. The withdrawal from LAAM has a delayed onset relative to methadone discontinuation but a similar time course (Sorensen et al. 1982). Buprenorphine, a partial μ receptor agonist with an extremely high receptor affinity (discussed later in this chapter), can also be used.

The noradrenergic approach to detoxification avoids the difficulties of prescribing an opioid to an addicted individual, but this method is less effective against many of the more subjective complaints during withdrawal, such as lethargy, restlessness, and dysphoria (Jasinski et al. 1985). The efficacy of clonidine in the treatment of opiate withdrawal in outpatients is controversial. A study (Gold et al. 1980) in which single doses of clonidine were compared with placebo in addicted subjects after methadone discontinuation showed that clonidine attenuated subjective symptoms such as nervousness, irritability, and subject ratings of opiate withdrawal. However, another study (Jasinski et al. 1985), in which clonidine was compared with placebo substitution in morphine-stabilized patients, found that clonidine attenuated many autonomic symptoms of withdrawal but had small effects on subjective withdrawal distress.

One very interesting pharmacological discovery is the ability of opiate antagonists to reverse opiate dependence and accelerate detoxification. Administration of naloxone in dependent monkeys has been found to cause desensitization to subsequent naloxone doses (Krystal et al. 1989). The use of an antagonist with another medication like clonidine to relieve the discomfort also seems to accelerate treatment in humans. Administering an antagonist such as naltrexone precipitates withdrawal within minutes for both methadone-maintained and ordinary heroin-addicted individuals, and this process of precipitation appears to decrease the duration of subsequent withdrawal symptoms. The amount of clonidine needed to ameliorate these symptoms when naltrexone and clonidine are used together is also lessened by using larger initial doses of naltrexone (Charney et al. 1982).

Recently, very rapid inpatient detoxification from opiates by using sedatives and anesthetics in combination with opiate antagonists has been reported. Loimer et al. (1990) reported a protocol involving barbiturate anesthesia with methohexitone (100 mg intravenous pretreatment, followed by 400 mg intravenously) and naltrexone (10 mg intravenously), which successfully detoxified patients from opiates in 48 hours. This procedure, however, required intensive medical treatment (intubation and artificial ventilation) and was accompanied by the risks of anesthesia and therefore is controversial. A subsequent study by this group (Loimer et al. 1991) with a similar strategy used midazolam, a short-acting benzodiazepine, to induce anesthesia, but this protocol nevertheless continues to require supervised administration of intravenous medication.

The long-term outcome of patients maintained on naltrexone after any detoxification essentially depends not on the induction process but on the strategies to retain them in treatment. If patients have a severe withdrawal reaction, they are not likely to be willing to stay on naltrexone. Relapse to illicit opiate use is frequent (usually over 90%) over a 6- to 12-month period without sustained outpatient treatment (Kosten 1990).

Another issue is that of "protracted withdrawal," which has been implicated in clinically crucial phenomena such as the difficulty of detoxification from methadone maintenance (Senay et al. 1977), high rates of relapse after abstinence (Dole 1972), and drug craving. Chronic use of opioids causes neurobiological alterations that persist for months after discontinuation of the opiates, although the phenomenon of protracted withdrawal is controversial. Up to 9 months after detoxification, opiate-addicted individuals manifest abstinence symptoms of weight gain, increased basal metabolic rate, decreased temperature, increased respiration, increased blood pressure, and decreased erythrocyte sedimentation rate (Martin and Jasinski 1969).

Longer-Term Treatments

Antagonist maintenance.   Antagonists should extinguish drug-seeking behavior by their ability to block the effect of narcotics. Naltrexone has a number of advantages over other opioid antagonists, including a relatively long half-life and an oral route of administration. The recommended dose of 350 mg per week can be administered daily, triweekly, or biweekly. It has no addictive potential and does not induce tolerance when used over long periods. Nevertheless, this "ideal" medication has not proved acceptable to most chronically opioid-dependent patients. The best results with naltrexone treatment have been reported in studies of physicians and other medical professionals or in structured settings, such as jail or work release programs, that provide a definite incentive for the maintenance of abstinence (Farren et al. 1997). However, in the less structured world of street addicts, treatment outcome for naltrexone was not considered successful: Only 50% of the patients were still taking naltrexone after 6 weeks, and only 10% of both the naltrexone group and the placebo group were doing so at 3 and 6 months.

Other than professional or institutionalized patients, possible suitable candidates for naltrexone include addicted patients early in their opiate abuse career or opiate-addicted patients with no previous treatment, individuals who have been abstinent but have recently relapsed, individuals who are currently abstinent but at risk for relapse, and individuals on a methadone program waiting list. Other strategies proposed to improve response to naltrexone treatment include payment or other positive incentives, such as an adaptation of the community reinforcement approach used in cocaine treatment (Farren et al. 1997).

Agonist maintenance.   Treatment of chronic opioid dependence is highly specialized and includes pharmacological as well

---

as psychosocial components. Methadone has long been the mainstay of the agonist treatment of opioid dependence and is a useful model for understanding the complex issues encountered in treating this population in general. Any discussion of that group of addicted individuals must be within this context.

Methadone is a safe, orally effective, long-acting agonist at the μ opioid receptor. Maintenance therapy with methadone is designed to support patients with opioid dependence for months or years while the patient engages in counseling and other therapy to change the opioid-dependent lifestyle. Although patients in methadone maintenance show physiological signs of opioid tolerance, there are minimal side effects, and patients' general health and nutritional status improve. Furthermore, investigators have shown that criminal behavior decreases in as many as 85% of maintenance patients, and employment typically ranges from 40% to 80%. Methadone maintenance programs are currently strictly licensed and regulated by the U.S. Food and Drug Administration and the Drug Enforcement Administration concerning the age (18 years) and the duration of dependence (at least 1 year) that are required of patients in order to qualify for this treatment.

Most clinics have a highly structured, behavioral mode of treatment with a major emphasis on rehabilitation. Explicit program goals include teaching patients real-life problem solving and enabling some program members to give up methadone. Many methadone programs are hierarchically structured, and rule making and rule enforcing are managed through a clearly defined chain of command. Clinics design their own rules and treatment programs within the guidelines set by state and federal agencies, and they vary with respect to the number of days open for dispensing, the number of take-home doses allowed, the number of urine toxicologies obtained, the intensity of behavioral treatment, and the doses of methadone used (Ball and Ross 1991).

Dose is a particularly important issue. When administered in adequate oral doses, a single dose of methadone in a stabilized patient usually lasts 24–36 hours without creating euphoria or sedation. Treatment staff have often tended to minimize maintenance doses because of the high value placed on abstinence in substance abuse treatment in general and concerns about the difficulty of detoxification from higher doses and diversion of medication to nonpatients. These concerns result in limits of 30- or 40-mg doses, which are clearly too low for many patients. Because narcotic cross-tolerance, or "blockade," is an essential therapeutic property of this medication in sufficient doses, patients should be given doses on an individual basis so that they have little chance of achieving an opioid effect from illicit drugs.

Scientific knowledge is now available to suggest that the original dosage protocol studied by Dole and Nyswander (1965) works best and that low doses are appropriate for only a limited number of patients. A series of large-scale studies has emerged showing that patients maintained on doses of 60 mg a day or more had better treatment outcomes than those maintained on lower doses (Ball and Ross 1991). The study by Ball and Ross (1991) revealed that opiate use was directly related to methadone dose levels; the effectiveness of methadone was greater for patients taking a 70-mg dose and was still more pronounced for patients taking 80 mg a day or more.

Methadone blood levels can also be affected by factors that have been demonstrated to significantly modify the metabolic breakdown of methadone in the body. These factors include 1) chronic diseases, including chronic liver disease, chronic renal disease, and possibly other diseases; 2) altered physiological states, particularly pregnancy (Chang 1997); and 3) drug interactions. The last factor included interactions of methadone with rifampin and phenytoin in humans and possible interactions with ethanol and disulfiram. In addition, by inference from animal studies, interactions may occur with phenobarbital, diazepam, desipramine, and other drugs, as well as with estrogen steroids, cimetidine, and antiviral agents used in the treatment of HIV infection (McCance-Katz et al., in press). These are described in more detail below.

Comorbid alcohol dependence introduces a special clinical challenge with respect to drug interaction problems. Alcohol is used to excess by 20%–50% of methadone-maintained patients and has a biphasic effect on drug metabolism (Kreek 1981). Disulfiram (Antabuse) is the only pharmacological agent available to methadone patients for prevention of alcohol abuse. It has been shown to date to have significant deterrent effects on recidivism after detoxification from ethanol. Although disulfiram also interacts with methadone metabolism, this does not appear to present a practical problem for treatment in most cases.

Psychosocial Aspects of Treatment

One of the major active research questions over the last several years has been the optimal intensity and type of treatment needed with respect to specific patient characteristics, treatment components, and outcomes. Only two prospective early studies of methadone efficacy, in which random assignment was used, were reported before the 1980s. Neither study focused on psychosocial treatment, but both studied methadone within the context of supportive treatment.

The first of these studies (Dole et al. 1969) used a relatively narrow range of outcome measures (relapse, employment, and crime). It did not describe the psychosocial treatment available to the control group but overwhelmingly supported the efficacy of methadone. In a second controlled, prospective study in Hong Kong (Newman and Whitehall 1979), 100 heroin-addicted volunteers were randomly assigned to groups receiving either methadone or placebo. All were provided with a broad range of supportive services. After 32 weeks, only 10% of the control subjects remained in treatment, whereas 76% of the methadone group continued and had less than half as many convictions for criminal activity than the control patients. Both of these studies agreed in that they found that methadone treatment was effective.

The most extensive and complete early review of methadone treatment is found in a study carried out by the National Institute on Drug Abuse (NIDA) (Cooper et al. 1983), which sponsored a series of meetings in which many aspects of methadone treatment, including outcome, were examined. Several large-scale studies had been completed and reviewed (McLellan et al. 1982). These studies confirmed that methadone-treated patients showed significant gains when compared with addicted subjects who were not in treatment. Documented improvements seen in methadone programs include reductions in illicit drug use and crime and increases in rates of employment.

These findings were further supported in a study by Ball et al. (1983) of treated and untreated addicted subjects in Baltimore and Philadelphia. These reports demonstrated significant reductions in criminal activity compared with equivalent time periods before treatment and were also verified by comprehensive arrest, penal, hospital, and other institutional data. This work was pioneering with respect to external validation of data and opened a doorway to matching subpopulations to elements of treatment other than to the pharmacological agent itself.

A second NIDA review (Grabowski et al. 1984) made another advance by attempting to further define specific patient characteristics with respect to the behavior problems demonstrated by addicted individuals and ways to manage those problems. The participants in this collaboration were in reasonably good agreement that it was essential for effective treatment programs to have a combination of support and structure involving specified rules that include suspension of those who display serious behavior problems.

As the effective use of methadone has become more clearly delineated, one specific question of importance for clinicians and clinical researchers is the efficacy of counseling services as an adjunct to methadone treatment for opiate-addicted patients. The need for such services has been questioned by some, leading to the promotion of methadone medication alone as a means of saving funds and including more patients in treatment.

McLellan et al. (1993) completed a prospective, random-assignment study of different levels of services within a methadone maintenance treatment program in order to examine this issue. In this study, volunteer patients were randomly assigned at the beginning of their methadone maintenance treatment to receive different types and amounts of treatment service over a period of 6 months. Level I patients received methadone maintenance (blocking doses of 60 mg or more) without additional counseling except on an emergency basis. Level II patients received the same methadone stabilization but also received regular counseling by a trained rehabilitation specialist. Level III patients received the same services as Level II patients but were also provided family therapy, employment, counseling, and regular medical and psychiatric services as needed.

The results of this study showed that patients in Level I experienced some improvement in drug use and modest improvements in employment but no other changes. The addition of a counselor to this level of services (i.e., Level II) was associated with significantly enhanced improvement in most areas. The additional services rendered by the family therapists, physicians, employment specialists, and social workers for Level III patients produced still more changes. Methadone alone therefore has some effects in patients with uncomplicated addiction, but substantial numbers of patients with additional disorders will not respond without the addition of other services.

Despite evidence for the effectiveness of psychosocial support, the actual trend has been a decline in these services, according to the 1991–1993 Drug Abuse Treatment Outcome Study funded by NIDA. Shepard and McKay (1996) performed a cost-effectiveness analysis of the study by McLellan et al. (1993), based on professional salaries, benefits, and number of contacts for patients in each group as prescribed by the protocol. Their analysis revealed that the intermediate level was more cost-effective ($16,150 per patient) than either the minimal level, which was least cost-effective ($22,558 per patient), or the high level ($19,969 per patient). A recently published follow-up on this study (Kraft et al. 1997) reported a similar relationship between cost-effectiveness of groups based on actual costs and outcomes at 6-month follow-up.

Another example of an even more intensive treatment is a day treatment program. To examine the hypothesis that a structured day treatment approach with methadone-maintained patients is more effective than standard treatment, we conducted an open pilot study. Patients admitted to the Veterans Administration (VA) Day Treatment Program between 1990 and 1992 ($n = 99$) were compared with a patient sample matched for sex (male) admitted to the inner-city methadone maintenance program at the APT (Addiction Prevention Treatment) Foundation in New Haven, Connecticut. The latter program offered only weekly therapeutic contacts during 1992 ($n = 89$) on the following outcomes: 1) illicit substance use during the first 3 months of treatment, 2) retention in treatment, and 3) employment status at discharge. The VA Day Program provided counseling, education, and recreation from 9:00 A.M. to 2:00 P.M. daily.

At the VA Day Treatment Program, a significantly smaller percentage of urine samples tested positive for illicit substances during the first 3 months of treatment than at the inner-city MMP site (21% vs. 55%, $P < .0001$). Patients' prospects for employment after participation in the VA Day Treatment Program were also improved: 49% of patients who were unemployed at admission to the VA program were employed at discharge, whereas only 4% were employed at discharge from the inner-city site.

This pilot study led directly to a recently completed study in which services on the upper end of the treatment intensity spectrum—a 25-hour-per-week day program—were compared with enhanced standard care. Both interventions were 12 weeks in duration, manual guided, and provided by Master's-level clinicians. Enhanced standard care consisted of standard methadone maintenance enhanced by the addition of a weekly skills training group and referral to on- and off-site services. There were no significant differences between the two interventions for opiate or cocaine use either during the 12-week treatment phase or at the 6-month follow-up. Over the course of treatment, drug use, drug-related problems, and HIV risk behaviors decreased significantly for patients assigned to both intensities (Avants et al., in review).

Ancillary Services and Special Populations

Concurrent Substance Abuse

Because it has not been clearly demonstrated whether agonist treatment itself promotes, attenuates, or has no effect on cocaine abuse, this treatment has been an ongoing subject of clinical research. Not only pharmacological but also psychosocial factors may play a role in the interactions between opioid substitution treatment and cocaine abuse. For example, methadone maintenance may facilitate cocaine use by freeing up time and money to buy cocaine that would otherwise have been used to buy opiates, by providing a high that is not dampened by methadone, and by being readily accessible to patients in the program (because it is often sold in the proximity of methadone maintenance programs). Mixing an opioid agonist like methadone with cocaine may prolong or even increase the euphoria with cocaine while attenuating the dysphoria afterward.

There are some limited preliminary indications that the dose of methadone may influence cocaine abuse in methadone-maintained patients. Some studies of cocaine use in methadone programs have indicated that methadone may place some patients at risk for increased cocaine use (Kosten et al. 1990). However, a pilot study (Stine et al. 1992) of an increasing-dose contingency protocol (in which the methadone dose was increased in response to positive cocaine toxicology) showed that 8 of 10 patients stopped cocaine use when they reached higher methadone doses of greater than 100 mg. This variable effect of methadone (i.e., entry into the program may increase use, but higher doses may decrease it) could be explained by the behavioral component of the contingency treatment described above. With the use of a pharmacological model, however, the results could also be explained by the differential effects of low and high methadone doses on the cocaine "high" or on cocaine-precipitated opiate withdrawal-like symptoms. One survey study (Stine et al. 1991) demonstrated that opiate-dependent patients do report cocaine-precipitated opioid withdrawal-like symptoms. A later study (Stine and Kosten 1994), in which low and high maintenance doses of methadone and buprenorphine were compared, confirmed greater symptoms of withdrawal in patients who used cocaine while maintained on the higher doses. There is some evidence that cocaine use is correlated to heroin use and that when methadone treatment is effective enough to decrease heroin use, decrease of cocaine use follows (Dunteman et al. 1992). These studies indicate an active, ongoing research interest in cocaine and methadone interactions. A larger, randomized dose-response study is needed to clarify the relationship of methadone dose to cocaine use. However, these results do call into question the practice of decreased methadone dose as a punishment for cocaine use.

The newer opioid agonist pharmacotherapies are now being investigated for possible therapeutic effects on cocaine abuse.

LAAM, the longer-acting methadone derivative, may prevent quick changes in opioid blood levels, which have been proposed to potentiate cocaine's effects (euphoria or "high") and increase abuse liability. For this reason, LAAM is also being studied for its effects on cocaine abuse in this population (A. Oliveto, personal communication, 1998). It has been suggested that buprenorphine, a partial opioid antagonist with relatively low opioid agonist activity (Jasinski et al. 1978; Kosten et al. 1993), may decrease the "speedball" interaction with cocaine and thereby reduce cocaine abuse. Three larger, controlled clinical trials produced conflicting results, showing no efficacy of buprenorphine over methadone in reducing cocaine abuse. Studies by Fudala et al. (1990), Kosten et al. (1993), and Schottenfeld et al. (1994) showed a dose-related reduction in cocaine use with buprenorphine. These studies are summarized below in the description of these new pharmacotherapy agents.

With increasing interest in alternative approaches to medical treatment in general, interest in acupuncture as a treatment for cocaine dependence has developed in recent years. Auricularacupuncture is a nontraditional form of acupuncture discovered by a French physician, Paul Nogier, in the 1940s. Theories concerning the mechanism of action of auricular acupuncture include modulation of neural circuits in the midbrain affected by drugs of abuse and stimulation of the vagus nerve in the auricle (Avants et al. 1997). Little empirical evidence is available for either of these theories, however. Auricular acupuncture specifically for the treatment of cocaine addiction has been employed for the last decade at Lincoln Hospital's Substance Abuse Division in Bronx, New York, and is reported to induce a state of relaxation and relieve withdrawal symptoms. More than 8,000 cocaine-abusing outpatients have received acupuncture treatments in this facility during this time, with approximately 250 patients treated daily (Smith 1991). Approximately 200 clinics offering auricular acupuncture for the treatment of addiction, including more than 20 methadone clinics, exist nationwide (Smith 1991). Despite this popularity, acupuncture has been evaluated in relatively few studies.

In an uncontrolled study conducted at Yale University, 32 cocaine-dependent, methadone-maintained patients received an 8-week course of daily auricular acupuncture, yielding an overall abstinence rate of 44%. Difficulty in identifying an appropriate control treatment has complicated research efforts. To date, four controlled studies have been conducted investigating the efficacy of acupuncture for the treatment of cocaine abuse. One randomized trial without an acupuncture control reported that cocaine-abusing subjects receiving acupuncture submitted significantly fewer cocaine-positive urines (21.8%) than did subjects receiving standard treatment plus frequent urine monitoring (28.3%). Three studies employed a needle puncture control, and all demonstrated no overall difference between the groups on percentage of cocaine-negative urines (Avants et al. 1997). Thus, although acupuncture has shown promise when compared with traditional drug treatment modalities, it has not been consistently shown to be more effective than a needle puncture control.

Medical Issues

HIV infection.   As described in detail in recent literature (O'Connor et al. 1994), infection rates among injection drug abusers in New York are high, yet the infection rate in the group of injection drug users in treatment is relatively low, making treatment of opioid dependence a clear public health need. However, despite risk reduction and prevention of new infection, there remains a need for treatment of an increasing number of existing HIV-positive, opiate-dependent patients.

Inner-city HIV-positive drug abusers need extensive medical and social services, which are most effectively delivered on site (Selwyn et al. 1993). Where this is feasible, the psychosocial intervention should include mechanisms for ensuring that on-site services are used appropriately. Where on-site delivery of medical and social services is not possible, it is essential to provide interventions for improving patients' compliance with medical regimens (e.g., keeping appointments and taking antiretroviral medications and prophylaxes against *Pneumocystis carinii* pneumonia and tuberculosis) and for connecting patients to community social service resources. Compliance with medical regimens has the potential to improve the quality and quantity of life and thus has an impact on motivation for changing high-risk behaviors.

The interactions observed among HIV infection, AIDS, and methadone treatment have led to the development of many specialized programs to provide research and deliver services in an attempt to manage the high numbers of infected patients. Special issues in the concurrent management of methadone and medications for HIV infection require integration of medical services for this population. These services include education about risk reduction by staff with special training in HIV spectrum disease, distribution of condoms, and assistance with referrals to infectious disease treatment services to determine the appropriateness of initiating antiretroviral therapy and to evaluate responses to therapy.

The introduction of new antiretroviral agents and the even more recent use of protease inhibitors have raised justifiable hope of a new therapeutic era for HIV-infected patients. However, this has also introduced new complexities in patient management, particularly for injection drug users, due in large part to potential drug toxicities and drug interactions.

The principal toxicities of the nucleoside analogues consist mostly of bone marrow suppression (zidovudine), peripheral neuropathy and pancreatitis (didanosine, zalcitabine, and stavudine, to varying degrees) and, less commonly, hepatitis (zidovudine, didanosine, zalcitabine) and diarrhea (lamivudine). Some of these toxicities may be particularly important in populations of HIV-infected drug users, in whom underlying rates of peripheral nerve disease, pancreatitis (due to coexisting alcohol abuse), and hepatitis (due to underlying alcoholic, drug-induced, or viral courses) may be very much higher than those in other HIV-infected populations (O'Connor et al. 1994). The metabolism of zidovudine is decreased by methadone, which may be associated with increased zidovudine toxicity (McCance-Katz et al., in press).

The principal toxicity of the non-nucleoside reverse transcriptase inhibitors (nevirapine, delavirdine) is rash. The protease inhibitors, in contrast, although very potent antiretroviral agents, can have significant side effects, including gastrointestinal distress (saquinavir, indinavir, ritonavir) and liver function and lipid abnormalities (ritonavir). Of the three available by prescription in mid-1995 (saquinavir, ritonavir, and indinavir), saquinavir and indinavir are generally better tolerated than ritonavir, but ritonavir may be the most potent of the three.

In addition to drug toxicities, there are important considerations regarding drug interactions: All the protease inhibitors are metabolized by the hepatic cytochrome P450 microsomal enzyme system and, to various degrees, may inhibit the metabolism of other drugs that are handled by this system, such as methadone and other opioids. This suggests that dose adjustments may be required, and in some cases certain medications may be contraindicated. Clinical and pharmaceutical studies are urgently needed to evaluate the possibly wide range of drug interactions for which HIV-infected drug users may be at risk by using this important new group of antiretroviral medications.

Liver disease.   In addition to the direct physiological effects of opioid use and abstinence, described above, there are a number of indirectly associated medical problems and problems resulting from both the direct and the indirect effects of opioid use. Chronic liver disease is the most common medical problem. Of all heroin addicts entering methadone maintenance, 50%–60% have biochemical evidence of chronic liver disease, primarily of two etiological types: 1) sequelae of earlier acute infection with hepatitis B or C virus, and 2) alcohol-induced liver disease including fatty liver, alcoholic hepatitis, and alcohol cirrhosis. Each of the major forms of viral hepatitis has been associated with injection drug use, hepatitis B and C being the most important.

A variety of studies have shown that over half of injection drug users are likely to show serologic evidence of past infection with hepatitis B virus (positive serologic test for hepatitis B virus surface and / or core antibody). A substantial proportion of this population also show evidence of active hepatitis B (hepatitis B surface antigen–positive) infection (O'Connor et al. 1994). These chronic carriers are at risk for transmitting hepatitis B infection and are more likely to develop chronic liver disease.

Hepatitis C virus is an important cause of posttransfusion hepatitis and of hepatitis among injection drug users (O'Connor et al. 1994). A variety of serologic studies of hepatitis C infection has found that, like hepatitis B, evidence of hepatitis C infection has been shown in the majority (more than two-thirds) of injection drug users. Hepatitis C is also associated with other causes of chronic liver disease, and there are three specific situations in which drugs may have hepatotoxic effects in these patients (O'Connor et al. 1994); these include 1) medications for the treatment of opioid dependence; 2) medications commonly prescribed to treat or prevent other infectious diseases associated with HIV or drug use, such as tuberculosis (isoniazid, rifampin) and opportunistic infections (trimethoprim-sulfamethoxazole); and 3) some antiretroviral agents (didanosine) (Kreek et al. 1976; O'Connor et al. 1994).

The bulk of severely chronically opioid-addicted patients in treatment receive methadone or other pharmacotherapeutic agents, and the liver plays a role in several aspects of the disposition of these medications. Nevertheless, methadone has been the most extensively and successfully used medication and has been well described as safe in milder disease.

Other infectious diseases. A variety of bacterial infections have been well documented to be associated with drug use in general and injection drug use in particular. Individuals with advanced HIV disease are at further risk for significant bacterial infections, including skin and soft tissue infection, pneumonia, endocarditis, and sepsis. In addition to bacterial infections, tuberculosis has long been known to be prevalent in drug users. The AIDS epidemic, however, has resulted in a major increase in the number of cases of tuberculosis (Selwyn et al. 1992). Often it is thought that tuberculosis in HIV-infected individuals represents reactivation of latent disease in the setting of immunosuppression, but it is also brought on by environmental and social factors related to drug use (O'Connor et al. 1994). HIV-infected individuals within the opiate-dependent population are at particularly high risk for extrapulmonary manifestations of tuberculosis (Braun et al. 1990), including infection of the gastrointestinal system or the CNS.

Psychiatric disorders. A large subgroup of opioid-dependent patients have psychiatric comorbidity. The inability to treat the psychiatric disorders of opiate-dependent patients contributes to poor treatment response and increased severity of all medical, addictive, and psychiatric problems of these patients. Studies have found that addicted individuals can have almost every psychiatric illness that occurs in nonaddicted individuals.

A comprehensive evaluation of psychiatric disorders in addicted individuals was completed by Rounsaville et al. (1982) in a sample of 533 opiate-addicted patients. In that study, depression was the most frequently diagnosed illness; about 60% of the sample had had some form of depression at least once. Alcoholism was the next most common problem, followed by antisocial personality and anxiety disorders. Schizophrenia, other types of personality disorders, mania, and hypomania occurred with a much lower frequency. Eighty-five percent of the patient samples were found to have had a psychiatric disorder in addition to opiate dependence at some time in their lives.

Many symptoms not systematically studied in the above report but also seen regularly are acute situational reactions involving intense but transient feelings of anger, anxiety, or depression; psychiatric disorders complicated by medical conditions such as hepatitis; and illnesses or injuries that produce chronic pain, such as pancreatitis, sickle cell anemia, or trauma resulting in nerve root irritation. Rounsaville et al. (1982) also found that untreated patients had similar types of psychiatric illnesses in relatively similar proportions to treated patients. However, treated patients were less likely to have a current psychiatric illness.

Women and Opiate Dependence

Opiate abuse and dependence in women has thus far defied facile treatment solutions. Available evidence indicates that most cases of opiate abuse and dependence in females is not treated and that it is more likely that the addicted female pursues medical treatment for the consequences of addiction rather than for the addiction itself.

Opiate-dependent women have higher rates of unemployment, depression, and anxiety disorders and more severe medical problems than do opiate-dependent men (Kosten et al. 1985). In the past, treatment services for opiate users have typically been based on research results focused on males, have served mostly males, and have been delivered by males. However, in the mid-1970s, with increased awareness of the treatment needs of women, treatment programs were designed to be more responsive by including more female staff members, limiting services to women, or taking child care responsibilities into account. Different types of programs attracted different types of women, although more women were likely to be retained in methadone maintenance programs than in therapeutic communities, which have been generally perceived to be less suitable for the female drug abuser (Chang 1997).

Copeland et al. (1993) compared 80 subjects from a residential specialist women's service and 80 subjects from two traditional mixed-treatment inpatient services in Australia. Both the specialist women's service and the mixed-treatment programs were based on the traditional disease model of addiction and the 12-step philosophy, but the specialist women's service employed only female staff and offered residential child care. The all-female staff and child care service were well received by female opiate abusers, but outcomes were no different. More research is needed to clarify which services are needed in order to improve outcome in women's programs.

Pregnancy is a special challenge in the treatment of opiate-dependent women. The potential medical and social costs of opiate dependence during pregnancy are great. Pregnant opiate-dependent women experience a sixfold increase in maternal obstetric complications and significant increases in neonatal complications (Dattel 1990). Pregnancy complications include low birth weight, toxemia, third-trimester bleeding, malpresentation, puerperal morbidity, fetal distress, and meconium. Neonatal complications include narcotic withdrawal, postnatal growth deficiency, microcephaly, neurobehavioral problems, and a 74-fold increase in sudden infant death syndrome (Dattel 1990). Treatment of pregnant opiate abusers has most frequently utilized methadone maintenance. Benefits conferred by methadone maintenance include removing the addicted woman from a drug-seeking environment, eliminating the need for illicit behavior to support a drug habit, and preventing fluctuations in maternal heroin level.

Chang et al. (1992) conducted a nonrandomized pilot study of an enhanced methadone maintenance program for addicted pregnant women that provided weekly prenatal care by a nurse-midwife, weekly relapse prevention groups, positive contingency awards for abstinence, and therapeutic child care during treatment visits. A randomized clinical trial comparing the enhanced program with regular treatment confirmed that neonatal outcomes from the enhanced programs were improved without affecting maternal drug use (Carroll et al. 1995). Subjects in the enhanced program had three times as many prenatal visits as control subjects and delivered heavier infants.

It is a commonly held belief that detoxification is difficult in heroin-addicted pregnant women and that maternal abstinence may cause fetal withdrawal in utero with a high risk of morbidity and mortality. Nevertheless, the controversial treatment option of opiate detoxification for these women has been raised for highly motivated women with extensive social supports or for those who may be entering long-term residential care after detoxification (Chang 1997).

In conclusion, the first generation of innovations in treatment for women, such as using female staff and limiting treatment to women, have been only partially successful. Specific efforts to tailor services to addicted pregnant women, such as adding prenatal care and child care, appear to improve pregnancy outcomes but do not reduce maternal substance use. The need for continued improvement remains, and this improvement may require addressing more difficult problems in these patients, such as the substance-abusing social supports that are frequently linked with addicted females and the greater likelihood that these women have histories of family dysfunction, sexual and other abuse, and untreated severe psychological or medical illness (Chang 1997).

The New Pharmacotherapies

LAAM

The 1993 approval by the U.S. Food and Drug Administration of LAAM for the treatment of opioid addiction represents the first and only opiate substitution alternative to methadone in more than 30 years of drug treatment. The pharmacological profile of LAAM is uniquely suited for the treatment of opiate-addicted individuals, and 40 years of clinical research have established its efficacy and safety in these populations. Fraser and Isbell (1952) first demonstrated the ability of LAAM to relieve symptoms of opiate abstinence and to serve as a cross-substitute for morphine by several routes of administration.

After oral administration, LAAM is well absorbed in the gastrointestinal tract. It is metabolized by sequential n-demethylation to nor-LAAM and dinor-LAAM. Both are potent opiate agonists, more potent, in fact, than the parent drug: The nor-LAAM is three to six times more active than methadone, and the dinor-LAAM is about equivalent to methadone. The combined pharmacological effects of LAAM and its active metabolites are greater after oral administration than after parenteral administration. After oral administration, the most intense opiate effects are observed within 90 minutes, reaching a maximum by 4 hours and persisting for approximately 72 hours (Fraser and Isbell 1952).

LAAM exerts its clinical effects in the treatment of opiate abuse by the same two mechanisms by which methadone is effective (Dole and Nyswander 1965). First, LAAM cross-substitutes for opiates of the μ agonist type, suppressing symptoms of withdrawal. Single doses of 30–60 mg of LAAM eliminate signs of abstinence for 24–48 hours. Second, repeated oral administrations of 70–100 mg of LAAM three times weekly produces cross-tolerance, which blocks the subjective "high" of subsequently administered heroin for up to 72 hours.

The clinical advantages of LAAM, both pharmacological and logistic, are related primarily to its slow onset and long duration of action. Because of the slow onset, there is less potential for abuse. In addition, because the medication is long acting and dispensed only from controlled programs, there is diminished potential for street diversion. Longer duration of action also provides a more consistent blood level and less fluctuation between doses. Logistically, less frequent dosing means less paperwork, less record-keeping, and less dose preparation time, enabling clinics to treat a larger number of patients. Thrice-weekly dosing also diminishes the need for take-home doses. Patients can be inducted directly onto LAAM from street heroin or can be transferred to LAAM after a period of methadone stabilization and maintenance.

The recommended starting dose for new patients is 20–40 mg. For patients already receiving methadone maintenance, most can transfer to LAAM at a thrice-weekly dose that is slightly higher than their daily methadone dose. The recommended initial dose of LAAM is 1.2–1.3 times the patient's current daily dose of methadone, not to exceed 120 mg. The history and current use of LAAM has been described in detail by Ling and Compton (1997).

Although the essential requirements for LAAM maintenance are the same as for methadone maintenance, special categories of patients may find LAAM particularly attractive. These include persons who rely on public transportation, those for whom employment or education schedules conflict with daily clinic attendance, and parents of small children (who are usually primarily single mothers). Additionally, some patients rapidly metabolize daily doses of methadone and report that it does not "hold" them for the entire 24 hours or that it causes unwanted acute sedation.

Buprenorphine

Buprenorphine, a derivative of the opium alkaloid thebaine (dimethyl morphine), is the newest medication currently being developed for agonist maintenance of opioid-dependent patients. It is metabolized in the body by both N-dealkylation and conjugation and has a terminal half-life of approximately 3–5 hours, but its opioid activity can be prolonged by administering high doses for 3 days (Rosen et al. 1994). Buprenorphine binds to all three types of opioid receptor, with an order of greatest affinity for $\mu \geq \kappa > \delta$ receptors (Sadee et al. 1982).

A unique characteristic of buprenorphine is that it dissociates very slowly from opioid receptor–binding sites (Hambrook and Rance 1976). It has been classified as a morphine-like (μ) partial agonist (Martin et al. 1976), producing ceiling effects on several measures and under some conditions blocking the effects of pure agonists. The larger the dose of buprenorphine that is administered, the longer is the duration of the antagonist effect. Ceiling effects are seen on respiration because buprenorphine produces an inverted U-shaped dose-effect curve (Doxey et al. 1977). Buprenorphine also elicits conditioned place preference with an inverted U-shaped dose-effect function (Brown et al. 1990), suggesting that it exhibits fewer reinforcing effects than either full agonists or other partial agonists.

Jasinski et al. (1978) were the first to examine the potential utility of buprenorphine as a treatment for opiate dependence in humans. Those authors showed that buprenorphine maintenance (8 mg/day, sc) attenuated the subjective and physiological effects of high doses of morphine (60–120 mg, sc) for up to 30 hours. A delayed withdrawal syndrome of mild severity occurred, suggesting that buprenorphine does not produce significant physical dependence in humans. Regardless of route, buprenorphine produced μ opioid agonist–like effects and miosis but no significant changes in respiration, body temperature, or cardiovascular measures.

When buprenorphine was abruptly terminated in these studies by Jasinski et al. (1978), the onset of withdrawal signs and symptoms was delayed by 1–14 days after placebo was substituted. The severity of withdrawal from buprenorphine when its administration was discontinued was greater than that from placebo but less than that from other opioid compounds, including morphine. As a maintenance agent, buprenorphine generally has a lower potential for physical dependence than other opioid compounds.

The optimal dosage regimen for buprenorphine has yet to be determined. Studies using daily maintenance doses as diverse as 1.5–16 mg (Kosten et al. 1991; Resnick et al. 1992) have consistently demonstrated treatment retention rates comparable to those for methadone maintenance therapy. Buprenorphine given sublingually at doses of 2 and 6 mg daily has been shown to be inferior to daily methadone doses of 35–65 mg on measures of retention in treatment, opioid-free urines, and self-reports of heroin use (Kosten et al. 1993). Johnson and North (1992), however, found that an only slightly higher dose of buprenorphine (8 mg daily) produced rates of heroin abstinence that were equivalent to those of methadone (60 mg daily). Dose-ranging studies (Bickel et al. 1988) have suggested that further increases in buprenorphine dose to as high as 16 mg daily may further improve abstinence from opiates.

A recently completed, large, multisite study (Ling et al., in review), supported by a collaboration of the VA Cooperative Studies Program and the NIDA Medications Development Division and designed for a labeling study for buprenorphine, will contribute to the clarification of dosing issues. Approval of buprenorphine as an agent for opioid maintenance medication is anticipated within 1 year of this writing.

Because of its long half-life, buprenorphine may be administered on an alternate-day or thrice-weekly schedule. Fudala et al. (1990) compared 8 mg of buprenorphine given daily with the same dose given on alternate days. Those authors found that only slightly greater opioid withdrawal symptoms were reported by subjects receiving buprenorphine on alternate days. Observations in outpatients have shown that patients receiving methadone doses of more than 35 mg daily are not likely to easily tolerate a transition to buprenorphine at 2–4 mg, sl (Kosten et al. 1989). For this reason, induction schedules for decreasing the methadone dose and gradually instituting buprenorphine must be used to transfer methadone patients to buprenorphine. Buprenorphine does not usually precipitate significant withdrawal symptoms in opiate-dependent individuals who are maintained at relatively low doses of methadone or who are using moderate amounts of street heroin.

Combined opioid and cocaine dependence occurs in up to 70% of heroin-addicted individuals, and more than 50% of these addicted individuals continue to use cocaine while in methadone treatment (Kosten et al. 1992). It has been proposed that a unique characteristic of buprenorphine is its ability to decrease the use of cocaine as well as of illicit opiates. Studies in nonhuman primates (Mello et al. 1989) that have been taught to self-administer cocaine showed robust dose-dependent decreases (60%–97%) in cocaine self-administration when these monkeys were treated with buprenorphine.

The effect of buprenorphine on cocaine use among opiate-addicted humans has been more equivocal. In the nonblinded study of Kosten et al. (1992), however, groups were not controlled.

In a double-blind, placebo-controlled study, Johnson and North (1992) compared buprenorphine, 8 mg/day, with methadone, 20 or 60 mg/day. Cocaine use was comparable in all subgroups at baseline, and there were no significant differences in cocaine use in any of the treatment groups. Schottenfeld et al. (1993), on the other hand, in a buprenorphine dose-ranging study (4–16 mg/day), found that subjects who were dependent on both opiates and cocaine significantly decreased their cocaine use with increasing doses of buprenorphine.

It has been theorized that buprenorphine has less diversion potential than methadone because it has combined agonist-antagonist effects. Although the potential of buprenorphine for abuse and dependence is much less than that of full opioid agonists, several instances of buprenorphine abuse have been reported (Pickworth et al. 1993), typically via the intravenous route—the user dissolves in water one or more 0.2-mg tablets intended for sublingual administration and injects the solution intravenously. A study in progress, also supported by Veteran's Administration Cooperative Studies Program (VA/CSP) and NIDA/Medication Development Division (MDD) ("A Multicenter Efficacy/Safety Trial of Buprenorphine/Naloxone for the Treatment of Opiate Dependence," Study 1008 A and B, co-principal investigators Peter Bridge and Paul J. Fudala, Ph.D.), is evaluating a buprenorphine-naloxone combination sublingual tablet that promises to further reduce the risk of diversion to intravenous abuse.

In summary, buprenorphine shows much promise as an alternative to methadone and naltrexone maintenance. It is well accepted by patients; has a mild withdrawal syndrome, which facilitates its discontinuation; reduces opioid and possibly cocaine abuse; and has greater safety and lower diversion potential than full agonists such as methadone.

Conclusions and Future Directions

Heroin-dependent patients are a heterogeneous group that may need relatively simple acute treatment, such as detoxification, or a complicated sequence of treatment interventions, beginning with high-intensity treatments and stepping down to much lower-intensity services over several years. Our most well-developed treatment intervention for chronic heroin dependence is clearly methadone maintenance, for which there is a wide range of ancillary approaches in addition to methadone itself. Optimizing methadone maintenance treatment can involve the use of other pharmacological agents in conjunction with methadone and the addition of a wide range of psychosocial interventions, from intensive day treatment programs to acupuncture. Medication alternatives to methadone, such as naltrexone, LAAM, and buprenorphine, have been increasingly available, and indications for matching to newly dependent patients and appropriate chronically addicted patients are developing.

The pharmacological and psychosocial tools available to us have vastly increased over the 30 years since methadone was introduced for the treatment of opiate dependence. The clinician needs to be aware of these alternatives for maintenance treatment as well as the advances in opiate detoxification in order to appropriately match patients' needs to these treatment alternatives.

References

Aghajanian GK: Tolerance of locus coeruleus neurons to morphine and suppression of withdrawal response by clonidine. Nature 267:186–188, 1978

American Psychiatric Association: Diagnostic and Statistical Manual of Mental Disorders, 3rd Edition, Revised. Washington, DC, American Psychiatric Association, 1987

American Psychiatric Association: Diagnostic and Statistical Manual of Mental Disorders, 4th Edition. Washington, DC, American Psychiatric Association, 1994

AT Forum: Smack is back—big time! Addiction Treatment Forum 6:1, 1997

Avants SK, Ohlin R, Margolin A: Matching methadone-maintained patients to psychosocial treatments, in New Treatments for Opiate Dependence, Vol 8. Edited by Stine SM, Kosten TR. New York, Guilford, 1997, pp 149–170

Avants SK, Margolin A, Kosten TR, et al: A randomized clinical trial of two intensities of adjunctive psychosocial treatment for unemployed methadone maintained patients: determining the optimal level of services (in review)

Ball JC, Ross A: The Effectiveness of Methadone Maintenance Treatment. New York, Springer-Verlag, 1991

Ball JC, Shaffer JW, Nurco DN: The day to day criminality of heroin addicts in Baltimore: a study in the continuity of offense rates. Drug Alcohol Depend 12:119–142, 1983

Bickel WK, Stitzer ML, Bigelow GE, et al: A clinical trial of buprenorphine: comparison with methadone in the detoxification of heroin addicts. Clin Pharmacol Ther 43:72–78, 1988

Braun MM, Byers RH, Heyward WL, et al: Acquired immunodeficiency syndrome and extrapulmonary tuberculosis in the United States. Arch Intern Med 150:1913–1916, 1990

Brown EE, Finlay JM, Wong JT, et al: Behavioral and neurochemical interactions between cocaine and buprenorphine: implications for the pharmacotherapy of cocaine abuse. J Pharmacol Exp Ther 256:119–125, 1990

Carroll KM, Chang G, Behr HM, et al: Improving treatment outcome in pregnant women: results from a randomized clinical trial. American Journal on Addictions 4:56–59, 1995

Chang G: Women and opiate dependence, in New Treatments for Opiate Dependence, Vol 10. Edited by Stine SM, Kosten TR. New York, Guilford, 1997, pp 190–198

Chang G, Carroll KM, Behr HM, et al: Improving treatment outcomes in pregnant opiate dependent women. Substance Abuse Treatment 9:327–330, 1992

Charney DS, Riordan CE, Kleber HD, et al: Clonidine and naltrexone: a safe, effective and rapid treatment of abrupt withdrawal from methadone therapy. Arch Gen Psychiatry 39:1327–1332, 1982

Cooper JR, Alterman F, Brown BJ, et al (eds): Research on the Treatment of Narcotic Addiction. Rockville, MD, U.S. Government Printing Office, 1983

Copeland J, Hall W, Didcott P, et al: A comparison of specialist women's alcohol and other drug treatment service with two traditional mixed sex services: client characteristics and treatment outcome. Drug Alcohol Depend 32:81–92, 1993

Dattel BJ: Substance abuse in pregnancy. Semin Perinatol 14(2):179–187, 1990

Dole VP: Narcotic addition, physical dependence, and relapse. N Engl J Med 286(18):988–992, 1972

Dole VP, Nyswander ME: A medical treatment for diacetylmorphine (heroin) addiction. JAMA 193:646–650, 1965

Dole VP, Robinson JW, Orraca J, et al: Methadone treatment of randomly selected criminal addicts. N Engl J Med 280:1372–1375, 1969

Doxey JC, Everitt JE, Frank LW, et al: A comparison of the effects of buprenorphine and morphine on the blood gases of conscious rats. Br J Pharmacol 60:118P, 1977

Dunteman GH, Condelli WS, Fairbank JA: Predicting cocaine use among methadone patients: analysis of findings from a national study. Hosp Community Psychiatry 43(6):608–611, 1992

Farren CK, O'Malley S, Rounsaville B: Naltrexone and opiate abuse, in New Treatments for Opiate Dependence, Vol 6. Edited by Stine SM, Kosten TR. New York, Guilford, 1997, pp 104–123

Fraser HF, Isbell H: Actions and addiction liabilities of alpha-acetyl-methadols in man. J Pharmacol Exp Ther 105:458–465, 1952

Fudala PJ, Jaffe JH, Dax EM, et al: Use of buprenorphine in the treatment of opioid addiction, II: physiologic and behavioral effects of daily and alternate-day administration and abrupt withdrawal. Clin Pharmacol Ther 47:525–534, 1990

Gallup GG, Suarez SD: Alternatives to the use of animals in psychological research. Am Psychol 40:1104–1111, 1985

Gold MS, Pottash AC, Sweeney DR, et al: Opiate withdrawal using clonidine. JAMA 243(4):343–346, 1980

Grabowski J, Stitzer M, Henningfield JE (eds): Behavioral Intervention Techniques in Drug Abuse Treatment. NIDA Research Monograph Series No 46. Rockville, MD, U.S. Government Printing Office, 1984

Hambrook JM, Rance MJ: The interaction of buprenorphine with the opiate receptor: lipophilicity as a determining factor in drug-receptor kinetics, in Opiates and Endogenous Opioid Peptides. Edited by Kosterlitz H. Amsterdam, Elsevier/North-Holland, 1976, pp 295–301

Jasinski DR, Pevnick JS, Griffith JD: Human pharmacology and abuse potential of the analgesic buprenorphine. Arch Gen Psychiatry 35:501–516, 1978

Jasinski DR, Johnson RE, Kocher TR: Clonidine in morphine withdrawal: differential effects on signs and symptoms. Arch Gen Psychiatry 42(11):1063–1066, 1985

Johnson SW, North RA: Opioids excite dopamine neurons by hyperpolarization of local interneurons. J Neurosci 12:483–488, 1992

Kosten TR: Current pharmacotherapies for opioid dependence. Psychopharmacol Bull 26(1):69–74, 1990.

Kosten TR, Rounsaville BJ, Kleber HD: Ethnic and gender differences among opiate addicts. Int J Addict 20:1143–1162, 1985

Kosten TR, Krystal JH, Charney DS, et al: Rapid detoxification from opioid dependence. Am J Psychiatry 146:1349, 1989

Kosten TR, Rounsaville BJ, Foley SH: Inpatient versus outpatient cocaine abuse treatments. Proceedings of the Committee on Problems of Drug Dependence, 1989. Rockville, MD, National Institute on Drug Abuse, 1990, pp 312–313

Kosten TR, Marby DW, Nestler EJ: Cocaine conditioned lace preference is attenuated by chronic buprenorphine treatment. Life Sci 49:201–206, 1991

Kosten TR, Morgan CA III, Falcione J, et al: Pharmacotherapy for cocaine-abusing methadone-maintained patients using amantadine or desipramine. Arch Gen Psychiatry 49:894–898, 1992

Kosten TR, Schottenfeld RS, Ziedonis D, et al: Buprenorphine versus methadone maintenance for opioid dependence. J Nerv Ment Dis 181(6):358–364, 1993

Kraft MK, Rothbard AB, Hadley TR, et al: Are supplementary services provided during methadone maintenance really cost-effective? Am J Psychiatry 154(9):1214–1219, 1997

Kreek MJ: Medical management of methadone-maintained patients, in Substance Abuse Clinical Problems and Perspectives. Edited by Lowinson JH, Ruis P. Baltimore, MD, Williams & Wilkins, 1981, pp 660–673

Kreek MJ, Garfield JW, Gutjahr CL, et al: Rifampin-induced methadone withdrawal. N Engl J Med 294:1104–1106, 1976

Krystal JH, Walker MW, Heninger GR: Intermittent naloxone attenuates the development of physical dependence on methadone in rhesus monkeys. Eur J Pharmacol 160:331–338, 1989

Ling W, Compton P: Opiate maintenance therapy with LAAM, in New Treatments for Opiate Dependence, Vol 11. Edited by Stine SM, Kosten TR. New York, Guilford, 1997, pp 11:426–466

Ling W, Wesson DR, Renner JA Jr, et al: Buprenorphine maintenance treatment of opiate dependence: a multicenter, randomized clinical trial. Addiction (in review)

Loimer N, Schmid R, Lenz K, et al: Acute blocking of naloxone-precipitated opiate withdrawal symptoms by methohexitone. Br J Psychiatry 157:748–752, 1990

Loimer N, Lenz K, Schmid R, et al: Technique for greatly shortening the transition from methadone to naltrexone maintenance of patients addicted to opiates. Am J Psychiatry 148:933–935, 1991

Martin WR, Jasinski DR: Physiological parameters of morphine dependence in man: tolerance, early abstinence, protracted abstinence. J Psychiatr Res 7:9–17, 1969

Martin WR, Eades CG, Thompson JA, et al: The effects of morphine- and nalorphine-like drugs in the nondependent and morphine-dependent chronic spinal dog. J Pharmacol Exp Ther 197:517–532, 1976

McCance-Katz EF, Jatlow P, Rainey PM, et al: Methadone effects on zidovudine disposition (ACTG 262). Journal of Acquired Immune Deficiency Syndromes and Human Retrovirology (in press)

McLellan AT, Luborsky L, O'Brien CP, et al: Is treatment for substance abuse effective? JAMA 247:1423–1428, 1982

McLellan AT, Arndt IO, Metzger DS, et al: The effects of psychosocial services in substance abuse treatment. JAMA 269:1953–1959, 1993

Mello NK, Mendelson JH, Bree MP, et al: Buprenorphine suppresses cocaine self-administration by rhesus monkeys. Science 245:859–862, 1989

Nestler EJ: Basic neurobiology of opiate addiction, in New Treatments for Opiate Dependence, Vol 2. Edited by Stine SM, Kosten TR. New York, Guilford, 1997, pp 63–118

Nestler EJ, Hope BT, Widnell KL: Drug addiction: a model for the molecular basis of neural plasticity. Neuron 11:995–1006, 1993

Newman RG, Whitehall WB: Double-blind comparisons of methadone and placebo maintenance treatments of narcotic addicts in Hong Kong. Lancet 8141:485–488, 1979

O'Connor PG, Selwyn PA, Schottenfeld RS: Medical care for injection-drug users with human immunodeficiency virus infection. N Engl J Med 331(7):450–459, 1994

Pickworth WB, Johnson RE, Holicky BA, et al: Subjective and physiologic effects of intravenous buprenorphine in humans. Clin Pharmocol Ther 53:570–576, 1993

Reisine T, Bell GI: Molecular biology of opioid receptors. Trends Neurosci 16:506–510, 1993

Reisine T, Pasternak G: Opioid analgesics and antagonists, in Pharmacological Basis of Therapeutics, 9th Edition. Edited by Hardman JG, Limbird LE. New York, McGraw-Hill, 1996, pp 521–557

Resnick RB, Galanter M, Pycha C, et al: Buprenorphine: an alternative to methadone for heroin dependence treatment. Psychopharmacol Bull 28(1):109–113, 1992

Rosen MI, Wallace EA, McMahon TH, et al: Buprenorphine: duration of blockade of effects of intramuscular hydromorphone. Drug Alcohol Depend 35:141–149, 1994

Rounsaville BJ, Weissman MM, Kleber HD, et al: The heterogeneity of psychiatric diagnosis in treated opiate addicts. Arch Gen Psychiatry 39:161–166, 1982

Sadee W, Rosenbaum JS, Herz A: Buprenorphine: differential interaction with opiate receptor subtypes in vivo. J Pharmacol Exp Ther 223:157–162, 1982

Schottenfeld RS, Pakes J, Ziedonis D, et al: Buprenorphine: dose related effects on cocaine-abusing opioid dependent humans. Biol Psychiatry 34(1–2):66–74, 1993

Schottenfeld RS, Kosten TR, Pakes J, et al: Buprenorphine vs. metha-
done maintenance for combined cocaine and opioid dependence.
Proceedings of the College on Problems of Drug Dependence, 1993.
NIDA Research Monograph Series 141:142. Rockville, MD, National
Institute on Drug Abuse, 1994

Selwyn PA, Sckell BM, Alcabes P, et al: High risk of active tuberculosis
in HIV-infected drug users with cutaneous anergy. JAMA 268:504–
509, 1992

Selwyn PA, Budner NS, Wasserman WC, et al: Utilization of on-site
primary care services by HIV-seropositive and seronegative drug
users in a methadone maintenance program. Public Health Rep
108:492–500, 1993

Senay EC, Dorus W, Goldberg F, et al: Withdrawal from methadone
maintenance: rate of withdrawal and expectation. Arch Gen Psychiatry 34:361–367, 1977

Shepard D, McKay J: Cost-effectiveness of substance abuse treatment.
Report submitted for U.S. Substance Abuse and Mental Health Ser-
vices Administration contract 271-89-8516. Waltham, MA, Brandeis
University, Center for Substance Abuse Treatment Research, 1996

Smith M: NIDA Newsletter, December 1991

Sorensen JL, Hargreaves WA, Weinberg JA: Withdrawal from heroin in
three or six weeks: comparison of methadylacetate and methadone.
Arch Gen Psychiatry 39:167–171, 1982

Stine SM, Kosten TR: Reduction of opiate withdrawal-like symptoms
by cocaine abuse during methadone and buprenorphine maintenance. Am J Drug Alcohol Abuse 20(4):445–458, 1994

Stine SM, Burns B, Kosten T: Methadone dose for cocaine abuse (letter).
Am J Psychiatry 148(9):1268, 1991

Stine SM, Freeman M, Burns B, et al: The effect of methadone dose on
cocaine abuse in a methadone program. American Journal on Addictions 1:294–303, 1992

Taylor JR, Lewis VO, Elsworth JD, et al: Yohimbine co-treatment during
chronic morphine administration attenuates naloxone-precipitated
withdrawal without diminishing tail-flick analgesia in rats. Psychopharmacology 103:407–414, 1991

Trujillo KA, Akil H: Inhibition of morphine tolerance and dependence
by the NMDA receptor antagonist MD-801. Science 251:85–87, 1991

Wise RA: The role of reward pathways in the development of drug dependence, in Psychotropic Drugs of Abuse. Edited by Balfour DJK.
Oxford, England, Pergamon, 1990, pp 23–57

Chapter 4

Substance Abuse and HIV Diseases: Entwined and Intimate Entities

Robert Paul Cabaj, M.D.

Introduction:
The Impact of Stigma and Prejudice

Medical professionals are taught to approach patients suffering from illness, sickness, and emotional concerns with compassion, objectivity, empathy, and hopefulness, providing interventions, treatments, support, and the alleviation of pain and suffering without morally judging the patient. It is ironic that the illness of substance abuse and alcoholism—so condemned and misunderstood by society, so layered with moralism and stigma—can provoke the same societally sanctioned negative responses in so many health providers. Criticizing patients because they use or abuse drugs, hoping to avoid working with substance abusers, refusing to recognize or to intervene with substance use or abuse, and minimizing the concerns of patients who acknowledge substance overuse or abuse are not uncommon reactions in mental health and health care providers.

Human immunodeficiency virus (HIV) is a retrovirus and presumably is like other retroviruses in having no moral codes or intellectual plan about how it goes about surviving and causing infection. HIV infection in humans has clearly been linked with causing acquired immunodeficiency syndrome (AIDS) and other AIDS-related and HIV-related conditions. HIV infection and AIDS provokes a response in the general public—and in many health care providers—that is similar to that elicited by substance abuse. The illnesses and infections may be labeled moral or sinful conditions, and some providers may try to avoid working with patients with HIV and AIDS and invoke moral arguments against them. The fact that HIV is spread through contact with infected body fluids—most commonly, semen during sexual activity and blood from shared needles for injection drug use—certainly contributes to this moralistic climate.

In addition, the demographic characteristics of patients with substance abuse disorders profoundly affect the ability of many of those who are HIV infected to obtain high-quality, consistent, and compassionate care. Women, gay men, members of ethnic minority groups, and people from deprived socioeconomic backgrounds may have limited access to unbiased and sensitive medical care and social services and may be distrusting of a medical establishment that has been perceived as prejudicial or uncaring. The stigma of having an HIV infection is compounded by the stigma attached to belonging to a minority group and is further compounded by the stigma attached to substance abuse.

Epidemiology

Substance abuse and HIV-related conditions are therefore intimately entwined through shared stigma and prejudice as well as through the routes of HIV infection. Sharing contaminated needles for injecting heroin, cocaine, amphetamines, or other drugs is the second-highest risk factor for HIV infection, according to the Centers for Disease Control and Prevention (CDC) (CDC 1997). Safer sex—behavioral interventions used to minimize the risk of HIV infection during sexual activity—works when the criteria are followed; however, when people who know about safer sex guidelines fail to follow them, most are intoxicated with alcohol or other drugs of use and abuse during, or just before, the sexual activity (as discussed below).

According to the 1997 CDC Mid-Year Surveillance Reports (CDC 1997), approximately 203,587 injection drug users (IDUs) have been diagnosed with AIDS nationwide to date. Injection drug use is a primary or secondary risk factor in 32% of AIDS cases—26% of IDUs plus 6% of IDUs and men who have sex with men (CDC 1997).

Comparable figures for substance-abusing, HIV-infected individuals who are not IDUs (such as those who are alcohol dependent or crack cocaine smokers) are less available. However, studies of drug use in high-risk groups, such as gay men, indicate very high rates of alcohol and drug use (Cabaj 1996).

Additional Cofactors to Consider

Working with HIV-infected substance abusers is not merely the sum of the parts, that is, working with the substance abuse aspects and working with the HIV-related aspects. The entwined and intimate nature of the two areas combine with many additional or cofactors that influence treatment.

Drugs and sexual activity.   Sharing HIV-contaminated needles clearly increases the risk of spreading HIV infection. More subtle, but extremely important, are the roles of alcohol, noninjected drugs of abuse, and abused prescribed medicines, which alter judgment and allow disinhibition of sexual behaviors. In most reviews of gay men and safer-sex practices, the great majority of men who were knowledgeable about safer sex failed to practice it while under the influence of some substance, such as alcohol or other drugs (Calzavara et al. 1993; Leigh 1990; Leigh and Stall 1993; Paul et al. 1994; Stall 1988; Stall et al. 1986).

In addition, some high-risk sexual activities that certain gay men enjoy—such as sadomasochistic interactions, activities such as "fisting" (the insertion of fingers, hand, or forearm into the anus and rectum of a partner), or attempts to extend and heighten the sexual experience—very often are done with the use of drugs such as amyl nitrite (known as "poppers"), alcohol, marijuana, and methamphetamine to help reduce inhibitions and induce physical relaxation (Cabaj 1985; Goode and Troiden 1979; Lange et al. 1988). Methamphetamine, also known as "crystal," "speed," "ice," or "crank," is especially dangerous as a risk cofactor. Besides being extremely addictive and used via needles or insertion in the rectum, the drug itself suspends all judgment and leaves the user often impotent but extremely sexually aroused and often an anal-receptive partner in sex (Gorman 1996; Gorman et al. 1995). Further, there is some evidence that most abused substances alter the immune system, which may well compromise the immune system's initial reaction to exposure to HIV in men engaging in unsafe sexual practices under the influence of such substances (MacGregor 1988).

In prevention efforts, focusing on just the activity that seems to be associated with the at-risk group, such as needle use for IDUs and safer sex for gay men, will miss the other routes of infection. Many IDUs have sex, are men who have sex with men, and use and abuse drugs.

Women.   Women are clearly at risk for HIV infection and are a significant portion of the people with AIDS in the United States. The CDC data noted above (CDC 1997) indicated that of a total of 612,078 AIDS cases nationwide, 96,075, or 15.7%, are in women. Of the 92,242 adult women with AIDS, 41,029 (44%) report injection drug use and 35,760 (39%) report heterosexual contact as their major risk factors. Of interest is the disproportionate share of AIDS cases among African American women—51,707 cases (56%) versus 21,319 cases among white women (23%) and 18,663 in Latina women (20%).

As discussed below, prevention efforts need to be custom tailored to the target population. Women from minority and underserved groups, especially those who are drug users, may have limited access to health care and messages about HIV risk reduction. Women with AIDS often have fewer social supports or help with their needs (Nyamathi et al. 1996). Women may be unaware of their HIV status and often learn of their serostatus when seeking help with a pregnancy or birth control.

Lesbians are clearly at risk for HIV infection, from both injection drug use and unprotected sex with men. Although it is still unclear whether infection via female-to-female contact can occur, lesbians have been urged to use safer-sex precautions such as dental dams during oral sex (White 1997).

Specific drugs of abuse.   Heroin (mostly injected), cocaine or crack cocaine (injected, intranasal, or smoked), and amphetamines (by various routes, including injection) are widely abused by HIV-infected substance abusers (Center for Substance Abuse Treatment 1995). In general, the most frequently abused substances in the United States are alcohol and marijuana, and they are so ubiquitous that patients may not even consider them as drugs of abuse unless specifically questioned about them during a substance abuse history.

Social and recreational use of drugs follows waves of popularity, and there are also regional phenomena and preferences particular to certain subpopulations. Lesser-known drugs may be used in certain groups. For instance, younger gay men in urban areas who use the "circuit" (a series of weekend-long parties that focus on dancing and sex) may be users of "party" drugs that include methamphetamine; MDMA (3,4-methylenedioxymethamphetamine), or "Ecstasy"; GHB (γ-hydroxybutyrate); ketamine; nitrate inhalants (poppers); and LSD (lysergic acid diethylamide) and other hallucinogens.

Performing interventions and establishing treatment plans for some drugs of abuse are easier than for others. For example, amphetamine abuse has been a problem for decades. Abuse of these drugs was nearly eradicated in the 1960s and 1970s as a result of a successful campaign initiated by the amphetamine-abusing community itself—the famous "Speed Kills" campaign that was effective when government-initiated campaigns failed. Nevertheless, there was a resurgence of amphetamine abuse in urban gay male communities and rural bikers in the late 1980s and 1990s, primarily because of its sexually enhancing effects (Baldinger 1996; Gorman 1994; Gorman et al. 1995; Munoz 1995; Sadownick 1994). Amphetamine abuse is particularly difficult to treat because the drug produces such euphoria and creates such a profound depression during withdrawal that users are prompted to use more of the drug to feel better. Many male streetworkers and young gay men are dependent on amphetamines, "tweaking" to have a sexual experience, and may exchange sex for drugs. Many purchasers of streetworkers are willing to pay a bit more money for unsafe sex, and many needy youths comply.

Crack, the more potent and concentrated form of cocaine, produces a similar picture and is a major drug of abuse among female streetworkers and adolescents from minority populations (Booth et al. 1993; Edlin et al. 1994). As with amphetamines, sex is exchanged for crack cocaine, often with little emphasis on safer sex.

Socioeconomic factors. Many substance abusers are from poor or limited economic backgrounds. Though gay men in general may be socioeconomically above the national average, gay chronic drug users may have lost their jobs or economic supports. HIV-infected people of color, both heterosexual IDUs and gay or bisexual men, may also be disenfranchised. Limited insurance, limited treatment options, and a limited ability to avail themselves of social services and enrollment in public assistance programs profoundly influence both the care of many HIV-infected substance users and the spread of the virus through limitations on education and outreach efforts. Minority status combined with substance abuse further limits access to care or makes patients wary about seeking care. Economic and societal forces often keep the minority substance abuser on the edges of society, with little hope of breaking out of settings that support easy drug or alcohol use, whether they be the "gay ghetto" created by homophobia or economic, geographic, and racial ghettos.

Overall Treatment Issues for HIV-Infected Substance Abusers

For the purposes of this chapter, *substance abuse* is defined as the inability to regulate the use of a substance in the face of problems with health, legal matters, work, and/or social life and relationships that are a result of, or concomitant with, the use of the substance. Substance abuse is marked by the loss of control over the use of a substance, usually including tolerance for the substance used—that is, craving or withdrawal symptoms when not using the substance—and a preoccupation with the substance used. Most abused substances alter judgment, cause acute and chronic changes in mental status, may affect memory and concentration, and may lead to chronic organic brain damage and possible medical problems from the use of the substances themselves or from the routes of administration—all major complications for HIV-infected patients that would be best to avoid.

Once a substance abuser has lost control over the use of the substance, he or she cannot return to controlled use; the loss of control is permanent. The goal of treatment for most substance abusers, therefore, is getting into "recovery," or learning to live clean and sober. Harm reduction models, described below, are approaches that attempt to limit the harm to a substance abuser before actually entering a treatment program. The most common and effective programs follow the 12-step models, and these models are the foundation of programs such as Alcoholics Anonymous (AA) and Narcotics Anonymous (NA).

Mental health providers need to understand the various substance abuse treatment modalities, ranging from the actual intervention when the substance abuser is confronted with his or her substance abuse and directed to a substance abuse treatment program, through early recovery with the help of 12-step or similar programs, to ultimate recovery, or living clean and sober. Outpatient medical and substance abuse treatment needs to be tailored to the ethnic, cultural, and sexual orientation status of the patient. If residential substance abuse programs are needed for treatment, housing, and linkages to care provision, a program that is familiar and comfortable with working with HIV-infected patients is recommended. Familiarity with and an understanding of the principle of 12-step recovery programs will enhance the medical care and the formulation of safe, adequate, and effective medical treatment plans for HIV-infected substance abusers.

Seeking and Entering Treatment: Interventions

The basic reasons that an HIV-infected substance abuser seeks and achieves recovery—that is, being clean and sober from drug and alcohol use—are enhanced quality of life, ability to help plan and cooperate with a medical treatment plan, enhanced compliance with and keeping of needed medical appointments and interventions, reduction of the use of emergency services, and reduction of the risk for opportunistic infections. The provider will face various types of substance-using patients seeking help or support for HIV-related concerns, most of whom fall into three broad categories: 1) those assessed to have a primary, untreated substance abuse problem; 2) those who will enter therapy or counseling and whose problems with substance use will be uncovered in the work; and 3) those who acknowledge a substance abuse problem and are in treatment but are seeking additional mental health support. The goals, needs, and challenges of each group can be very different.

Increasing numbers of HIV-infected patients were infected

through injection drug use or through unsafe sex that occurred under the influence of alcohol or other drugs. With this awareness, the mental health professional needs to recognize that many patients seeking help for HIV-related concerns will have a primary substance abuse problem that has not been diagnosed or treated. Very little can be done in conventional counseling, psychoeducation, or psychotherapy if the patient has active alcoholism or other substance abuse. The goal of most clinical interactions with such HIV-infected patients is to talk about risk factors and risk-reduction behavior when the patient is not intoxicated. Even if they are somewhat intoxicated, these patients may be able to comprehend HIV risk factors, in the hopes of reducing the spread of HIV (harm reduction). In addition, it should be emphasized to the patient that the substance abuse is a problem in itself that needs to be reduced and/or treated.

Several models exist to understand substance abuse, including psychodynamic, disease, social, and moral models. In the disease model, the abuse is seen as an illness that may have genetic and biological factors that may be influenced by cultural and social stressors. In this model, the disease of substance abuse is manifested by the loss of control over the use of the substance, followed by concomitant problems as described above.

The fact that the hallmark defense mechanisms of most addicted persons are denial, projection, and fear of suffering makes treatment challenging, but quite possible. Using the disease model, there is no guilt or judgment about drug or alcohol use; loss of control is understood, and the impossible challenge to cut down and limit use is avoided. The goal of living clean and sober, completely free of all alcohol and drug use, is underlined. Relapse, or the episodic return to drug or alcohol use, is seen as a part of the disease and ongoing recovery process, not a treatment failure. Traditional psychotherapy is not effective for the treatment of substance abuse but might help prepare a patient for such treatment.

A common belief among treatment providers is that patients do not see that they have a substance use problem or need to get into recovery until they have "hit bottom," or have recognized that their lives have fallen apart and have reached the lowest point. Providers performing the initial assessment can help "raise bottom," that is, help patients see that the substance-abusing path they are taking will lead to worse problems. The knowledge of having an HIV infection can often be the turning point for such patients, an important opportunity to plant the seed of awareness of the need for recovery and learning to live clean and sober.

Substance use and abuse do not in and of themselves prevent proper treatment of the HIV-infected person. The provider needs to perform a proper assessment and match the patient with the services that will be most beneficial. Although actively using substance abusers are not good candidates for psychotherapy or insight-oriented groups and educational efforts, they may benefit from support and educational groups that are experienced in working with substance users. HIV-infected patients who use recreational drugs but are not addicted may benefit from reduction in use and can also benefit from psychotherapy, support groups, and educational efforts. Providers need to remember that increased stresses or medical changes and setbacks may lead to relapse in the abuser in recovery and may also influence the ability to use mental health services.

Although a few substance-abusing patients may react to the knowledge of their HIV status with feelings of hopelessness and may plunge into increased alcohol or substance abuse, my experience is that, after the initial shock and adjustment period, most substance abusers wish to have a working knowledge of HIV and health factors, as well as information about risk factors to prevent infecting others. A discussion about the detrimental effects of substance use and abuse on health care in general and HIV progression in particular, as well as the ill effects of the disease of substance abuse itself, leads many substance abusers to seek help with their substance use. Interventions—that is, finding treatment programs or formulating intensive treatment plans for the substance abuse—are common at this point.

Assessments

Many HIV-infected patients have experienced prejudice or stigmatization by the medical community and may be inhibited in talking about even casual substance use. They may assume that the provider will judge them negatively and thus may not talk about, or may minimize, their substance use in order to be more accepted by the provider. Denial is also a major part of substance use and abuse and further contributes to limited information sharing.

An assessment of and discussion about substance use is essential for working with HIV-infected patients for several reasons:

1. As described above, there may be a lapse into higher-risk sexual behavior with drug or alcohol use.
2. The abuse of alcohol or other drugs will interfere with understanding the nature of HIV infection and the necessary medical and psychosocial care.
3. Drug or alcohol use and abuse may cause direct medical harm, and the patient may be at higher risk for infections, especially tuberculosis.
4. Continuing use and abuse may lead to rejection by loved ones, families, or even the health care system.
5. A thorough assessment of substance use will help with the proper educational efforts and referral for the best type of counseling or therapy.

An assessment for substance use or abuse should occur as early as possible in the evaluation of a new patient. Ideally, such an assessment would be part of an initial intake, incorporated into the usual psychosocial and psychiatric assessment to avoid making it an isolated issue. Questions about drug or alcohol use can be asked in the same matter-of-fact, nonjudgmental way in which questions about sexual orientation and sexual practices are asked. If these questions are seen as part of a risk assessment and psychosocial assessment, the patient is more likely to give accurate information. Questions to ask or information to obtain (which can expand or contract based on the individual's history, or if the patient seems defensive or avoidant around the subject of alcohol or drug use) include the following:

- Describe most recent drug and alcohol use.
- Is there current or past intravenous or injection drug use?
- What is the frequency of drug use and setting for use?

- Which is the "drug of choice," that is, the drug the patient enjoys or seeks most?
- Has the patient felt guilty or concerned about drug or alcohol use, or does the patient believe there is a problem with the drug or alcohol use?
- Does anyone close to the patient believe there is a problem?
- Have there been any problems with health that might be related to the use of alcohol or other drugs?
- Has the patient had legal problems due to drugs or alcohol, including driving under the influence?
- Has the patient undergone financial or employment problems related to the substance use?
- Has the patient had social problems or lost lovers, family, or friends related to use?
- Has the patient had treatment in the past for substance abuse? If so, what type of treatment, and when?
- What is the longest period the patient has refrained from drug or alcohol use?
- What did the patient do to stay "clean and sober," that is, free from drug and alcohol use, during that period?

The evaluator may expect some anxiety or resistance to these questions, especially if the patient has had concerns about substance use, and may not be able to get all the information needed in the first visit. In fact, for many patients, the actual pattern of substance use and the impact it has on their lives may not become clear until they have been in treatment for some time.

A more detailed drug and alcohol history can be taken when indicated, including specific drugs used, age at first use, and more detailed problems or treatment related to substance use. If it is clear that the patient is a substance abuser and would like help, traditional psychotherapy is not indicated; referral to an appropriate substance abuse treatment program or provider would be best.

Mental health and medical care should not be cut off if a patient refuses to get into recovery. An altered form of a full-scale intervention can be helpful, listing the symptoms and evidence that the provider sees to support the diagnosis of substance abuse, as well as the probable problems ahead if something is not done to treat it. Many patients with HIV infection and substance abuse have used the infection as the inspiration to get into recovery, hitting bottom before experiencing the total legal, social, medical, and employment failures that many people need to experience before getting into recovery.

Treatment Programs and Harm Reduction

Substance abuse treatment on demand is an ideal achieved in only a few communities. The limited availability and access to treatment programs, or "slots" in treatment programs, interfere with the total care of the substance abuser. These limitations are due to fiscal limitations as well as to political and community influences. Politicians are still hesitant to support substance abuse treatment for fear that taking such a stand will be seen as condoning substance use. Local communities often resist the establishment of treatment programs—the "not-in-my-neighborhood" mentality. In many communities, the limited treatment slots that are available may be saved for HIV-infected patients, making HIV-infection prevention efforts even more difficult.

Overwhelming evidence supports clean needle exchange in dramatically reducing the spread of HIV among IDUs (Lurie 1993; Ostrow 1994). Most localities, however, outlaw or limit the availability of clean needles, again primarily for political reasons. The federal government's own studies support the beneficial impact of clean needle exchange (Lurie 1993), yet the U.S. Department of Health and Human Services will not take a stand supporting the establishment of clean needle exchange programs nationwide. The President's National AIDS Council has threatened to resign over the refusal to back the prevention of HIV infection that is inherent in needle exchange programs.

The substance abuse treatment community itself is divided on the importance and impact of methadone treatment programs for opiate-addicted individuals. Although methadone has been clearly demonstrated to reduce the spread of HIV, reduce crime related to seeking money for drugs, and allow the opiate-addicted individual the opportunity to return to employment or other socially beneficial activities, methadone is often criticized for being just an "addiction substitute" rather than a true path to recovery (Novick and Joseph 1991). In addition, the same political influences noted above influence the establishment and support of methadone treatment programs.

Substance abuse treatment professionals may also inadvertently present barriers to treatment, especially if they insist that patients be totally abstinent from drug and alcohol use before they enter treatment. Providers and programs who are able to tolerate the patient who is seeking help but who has not yet been able to achieve sobriety are those most likely to engage the patient who is interested in getting help for both HIV and substance abuse.

An increasingly popular model is a combination of the harm reduction and relapse prevention models of intervention (American Medical Association 1996; Brettle 1991; Fernandez and Levy 1994; Springer 1991; Strang 1992). Sobriety and recovery are always the ultimate goal, but realistic steps along the way to that goal are promoted, such as cutting down on use, encouraging the use of clean needles, promoting safer-sex guidelines, and identifying situations that trigger substance craving and employing a type of behavior modification to avoid these situations (relapse prevention). Even if not every single instance of sexual contact or needle sharing is safe, every reduced-risk encounter is a harm reduction event. Every time drugs and alcohol are not used when they would usually be used, better judgment, awareness, or even recovery may follow.

Medical Management and Social Needs

The acute and chronic sequelae of substance abuse greatly complicate the assessment and treatment of HIV-related medical concerns (Sorenson and Batki 1992). In addition, many health providers assume that drug users are indifferent about their health and will not comply with treatment recommendations, leading to lower standards of care for this population. There are some specific situations in which the clinical impact of the drug of abuse must be dealt with first.

The intoxicated patient. In providing care for HIV-infected substance abusers, the first concern is to ensure the patient's immediate safety. An HIV-infected person who appears drunk, for example, may have altered mental status due to various possible causes, including medication side effects or life-threatening infections of the central nervous system (CNS). If it is clear that the patient is indeed intoxicated, a brief discussion and a request to return when he or she is not under the influence is most helpful. If a patient repeatedly shows up intoxicated, it is important to let him or her know verbally, and preferably in writing, that this is unsafe and that increased efforts will be made to link that person with substance abuse treatment so that he or she will be more likely to benefit from each mental health or medical visit.

Withdrawal from drugs of abuse can create a clinical picture that mimics numerous complications of HIV. Inpatient admission may be necessary for complicated withdrawal from alcohol or other drugs. Patients who have advanced AIDS, are pregnant, or are in any way medically unstable may require inpatient admission. Patients with acute psychiatric conditions, especially suicidality or psychosis, usually require medically supervised detoxification.

Alcohol and other central nervous system depressants.   Drugs that depress the CNS, such as alcohol, present the greatest danger in withdrawal. These hazards include seizures, autonomic instability, aspiration pneumonia, and the many sequelae of delirium. Benzodiazepines are the safest and most studied class of medication used for the treatment of withdrawal from CNS depressants. Usually, long-acting agents such as chlordiazepoxide or diazepam are preferred. If liver functioning is a concern, lorazepam or another nonhepatically metabolized benzodiazepine can be used. Other options for detoxification include phenobarbital, valproic acid, and carbamazepine.

Opiate withdrawal.   Although rarely life threatening, opiate withdrawal can be extremely uncomfortable and debilitating and needs to be addressed. The symptoms of opiate withdrawal (elevated pulse and blood pressure, nausea and diarrhea, sweats, pain) can needlessly confuse diagnostic workups and may compromise a patient's ability to comply with treatment (Selwyn 1989).

If a methadone clinic is available, providing methadone is the best option because it usually allows a 21-day detoxification and some provision for connecting the individual to longer-term treatment. When this is not possible, opiate withdrawal can be treated symptomatically with clonidine (often initiated at 0.1 mg three times daily and titrated up as needed) with the addition of analgesics such as ibuprofen, diphenhydramine (Benadryl) for sleep, and agents for diarrhea. For patients taking multiple medications, it is important to note that phenobarbital, phenytoin (Dilantin), carbamazepine, and rifampin (and probably rifabutin) can drastically lower blood levels of methadone. Protease inhibitors can raise methadone levels.

Adherence and noncompliance. In the earlier years of the HIV epidemic, HIV specialists had a patient population primarily composed of gay, middle-class, white men. Many of these could be classified as "ideal" patients who appeared promptly for appointments, took medications as prescribed, and educated themselves about their illness. Most such patients were extremely active in their own treatment decisions and day-to-day care and had the support of friends and lovers. As the demographics of the HIV-infected population have changed, providers are now challenged with drug-abusing patients who may not be able to comply with treatment as easily. Studies have shown that AIDS-diagnosed IDUs, women, and minorities are significantly less likely to receive zidovudine than are other AIDS-diagnosed patients (Johnston et al. 1994). This could be a reflection of access to treatment and economic concerns, but in assessing IDUs who were actually prescribed zidovudine, a survey showed that over half had significant difficulties in adhering to the medication regimen (Wall 1995). Comorbid mental illness also interferes with adherence (Ferrando et al. 1996).

In some patients, obstacles to taking medication may be overlooked. Often these patients have practical survival concerns related to their housing and finances. For a person who is homeless or in transitory housing, medications are easily stolen or lost. Without a watch, he or she may not be able to take the medication on time. Transportation to the clinic may be unaffordable. Just surviving on the street for the next week is much more terrifying than abstract concerns about future health problems.

The use of protease inhibitors, the best treatment in combination with other antiviral agents for people with AIDS to date, requires strict adherence on a set time schedule. A preliminary study at San Francisco General Hospital showed a significant failure rate of protease inhibitors that in many cases was attributable to noncompliance in substance abusers (San Francisco Chronicle 1997a). Other preliminary studies, however, support the fact that substance abusers can follow the medication guidelines, especially with case management, as discussed below (Barthwell 1997; San Francisco Chronicle 1997b).

A coherent plan and a continued effort for adherence , including the use of case management, must therefore be made for HIV-infected substance abusers. It may be necessary to use the assistance of visiting nurses or to place the person in a structured living setting where medications are administered daily. A methadone clinic might elect to administer HIV medications with the daily methadone dose (Selwyn 1989), although this approach is at best only a partial solution because most HIV therapeutic agents are given in multiple daily doses.

Case management for HIV-infected substance abusers. Case management has long been a tool in social work and was developed for working with the chronically mentally ill. The case management approach to HIV-infected substance abusers must differ from that traditionally used, given the nature of substance abuse and the risks of HIV infection.

Routine case management consists of helping patients learn about services and helping them to negotiate through or around the many barriers and obstacles to services. This approach is effective when the patient is motivated, has some ability to care for himself or herself and to use adequate judgment, and has a relatively stable social environment from which to negotiate. Intensive case management may be more helpful for the severe substance abuser and includes direct outreach, assistance in keeping appointments, advocacy for medical and social services, direct assistance in applying for public support, assistance in taking medications, and brokering directly for admission to substance abuse services (rather than leaving it up to the patients to try and negotiate it all for themselves) (Nix and Cabaj 1992).

Prevention Efforts

Substance abuse treatment is HIV prevention! This sentence is the newest way of approaching the demographic changes in the AIDS epidemic (Shoptaw and Frosch 1997). As the number of IDUs with AIDS and HIV infection continues to increase, the intimate role of the two conditions is the focus of prevention. More efforts are needed to target the population of drug and alcohol users who are not yet HIV infected. Increased access to treatment and better distribution of limited treatment slots for both HIV-positive and -negative patients is needed for true prevention efforts.

Literature and ad campaigns targeted for specific audiences are crucial for HIV prevention. Literature that is appropriate for gay men will not be effective for African American IDUs in the inner city; Latinos who are monolingual in Spanish will not benefit from the clean-needle literature if it is presented only in English. Women have needs that are very different from those of men and that should be addressed. Lesbians are very much at risk for infection, through either needle use or sex with HIV-infected men, and need their own targeted prevention efforts.

Going to where the at-risk people are, as opposed to hoping they will chance upon the prevention efforts somewhere along the way, continues to be the most reasonable trend in prevention efforts. HIV and AIDS awareness groups are targeting gay bars and giving out condoms at the exits. Advertisements are focused on bisexual people of color. Campaigns in which someone declares, "I always follow safer sex guidelines . . . until my third drink," as well as others, explore the link of alcohol and other drugs with sex. The Center for Substance Abuse Treatment insists that all substance abuse treatment programs have guidelines for the treatment of HIV-infected individuals and add prevention efforts (Center for Substance Abuse Treatment 1995).

As discussed above, needle exchange is a form of HIV prevention. The harm reduction approach as well as the relapse prevention models are also prevention models. Education of the patient and his or her responsibility can be an integral part of treatment and also supports prevention efforts.

Understanding the links between substance use and HIV risk behaviors has been the subject of many studies and reviews (Ostrow 1997; Ostrow and McKirnan 1997). The research still supports the contention that the gay men who become HIV infected now are more likely to be substance users and abusers. Efforts to break this link therefore need to be a part of prevention efforts (Ostrow 1996; Stall 1997). Specific subgroups, such as Latino gay men, have also been studied to understand the link between sex and substance use (Diaz and Ayala 1997).

Mental Health Treatment and Psychotherapy Issues

Once an HIV-infected substance abuser is in treatment for mental health, medical, and/or substance abuse problems, several long-term issues arise related to ongoing care and attempts to achieve sobriety. The ideal treatment would involve a close alliance and consultation with all the providers involved, especially the psychiatrists and physicians who might be prescribing medications. Some basic issues have already been mentioned: recognition that a relapse or return to substance use is always possible in a patient in recovery; and that stressful events in life, such as financial losses, changes in health, the death of a friend or lover, or even awaiting HIV serostatus testing results, increase the risk of a relapse.

Gay men and lesbians may need a treatment program that is specifically targeted to their needs, because homophobia, both internalized and experienced from society, is a significant force leading to substance use, as described below. Treatment for women with children needs to allow for child care for those mothers who cannot arrange such care. People of color with HIV and substance use concerns may not feel comfortable attending a treatment program in a hospital, clinic, or more traditional setting that is not always welcoming to minorities, and instead might benefit from services provided in the local community, such as at churches or schools.

Psychopharmacology

Clearly, many prescribed medications can be abused and might potentiate a relapse in an abuser who is clean and sober. Minor tranquilizers, such as the benzodiazepines, are easily abused and may facilitate an alcoholic patient who is in recovery to start drinking again. Stimulants used to treat depression can clearly be abused and may cause relapse in an amphetamine or cocaine abuser. Pain medications, which are often needed for a variety of acute situations or for chronic pain management, may lead to relapse in an opiate abuser.

Anxiety. Adjustment disorders are the most common anxiety disorders in HIV-infected patients, and panic disorders may present more often in these individuals than in the general population. Symptoms of anxiety may be the ones that providers can most easily treat with psychopharmacology, which may help explain the vast amounts of antianxiety agents prescribed—and abused. Most anxiety can be treated, however, without medications. Attentive listening and concern on the part of the provider, education and direct answers to questions, rapid decision making and turnaround of test results, and simple basic counseling may serve to relieve the anxiety that is due to situational concerns and reactive conditions. Biofeedback, acupuncture, self-hypnosis, meditation, and behavioral interventions all have a role in treating anxiety.

The medications used to treat anxiety are, for the most part, quite safe, produce minimal side effects, and present little danger from overdose. Possible contraindications for the use of the most common category of antianxiety agents, the benzodiazepines, are a diagnosis of primary alcohol and substance abuse; moderate to severe dementia, because benzodiazepines may cause confusion and memory loss; and severe nonagitated depression, because benzodiazepines may themselves cause depression with chronic use. Benzodiazepines work best when used for only short periods for the acute management of severe anxiety. Tolerance is easily developed, especially with daily use at even low to moderate doses. Patients may seek increasing doses if they use the medications on a regular, daily basis, rather than as needed and with a break of a few days between use. All benzodiazepines require careful tapering to stop after continued use. Abruptly stopping a chronically used benzodiazepine may trigger a prolonged withdrawal state ranging from insomnia, anxiety, and a flulike state to seizure and delirium, like delirium tremens resulting from abrupt alcohol cessation.

Buspirone (Buspar) is an alternative to the benzodiazepines. It is not sedating, has few if any cognitive side effects, and does not create dependency or addiction. The major drawback of this drug is the long period—up to 4 weeks—required before it takes effect. Some patients report no effect from this medication, and most patients used to benzodiazepines will not tolerate the waiting period (Batki 1990a). Acute anxiety might need to be treated concurrently with benzodiazepines when buspirone is prescribed; the benzodiazepines can then be tapered and stopped within 2–4 weeks. Alternative psychopharmacology mainly exploits the side effects of other medications, such as the sedating effects of antidepressants or antihistamines, rather than having a primary effect. These alternatives should be considered only when benzodiazepines or buspirone is not indicated.

Insomnia.   Insomnia is one of the most common symptoms in HIV-infected patients. It can have many causes and may be an indication of an undetected but treatable depression (Perkins et al. 1995). Hypnotic benzodiazepines are most commonly prescribed for insomnia, but again, all the comments about the benzodiazepines apply. For a substance abuser in whom benzodiazepines may be contraindicated, the best sedating agent to consider is the antidepressant trazodone (Desyrel and others). Although not a very potent antidepressant, trazodone is very sedating and is an excellent, nonabusable agent to help with sleep.

Depression.   Depression is the second most common reason for mental health assessment and intervention for HIV-infected patients. Sadness, grief, fear, demoralization, and bereavement may all appear as depression and may all be healthy and normal reactions to losses that the patient has experienced or anticipates. A careful assessment and diagnosis are therefore necessary.

Although psychopharmacology may be indicated for diagnosed mood disorders, nonpharmacological interventions may also be indicated. Individual psychotherapy may be quite effective, without medication side effects (Markowitz et al. 1995). Supportive or intensive group therapy can be extremely useful and can not only help patients with presenting symptoms but can also provide some ideas and guidance in negotiating the course of the HIV illness.

When antidepressants are used, lower doses than usual may be indicated, due either to the sensitivity exhibited by HIV-infected individuals or to the combination of other medications a patient may be taking. In general, antidepressants, except for the psychostimulants, are not addicting and can usually be safely used in substance abusers.

Antidepressants fall into several major categories. The most common are the traditional tricyclics and the newer serotonin-specific reuptake inhibitors (SSRIs). Some newer categories are being discovered and made available for use, but these have had little studied use with HIV-infected patients. A broad category of antidepressants, the monoamine oxidase inhibitors, have little or no role in treating HIV-infected patients because these drugs have too many dangerous interactions with other medications and certain types of food.

Although imipramine has been noted to help depressed patients with HIV illnesses (Rabkin et al. 1994a), most tricyclic antidepressants have significant anticholinergic side effects. The SSRIs are the safest antidepressants to use, both in terms of side effects and lethality if used in overdose, and are the easiest to prescribe and monitor for side effects. Compliance in general is better with the SSRIs than with the tricyclics.

Sertraline (Zoloft) may be the SSRI of first choice; it is well tolerated, has the least effect on hepatic enzymes, and is the least stimulating among the SSRIs (Rabkin et al. 1994b). The other SSRIs are equally effective and may be exploited for their somewhat more energizing side effects in patients who present with extreme loss of energy. Fluoxetine (Prozac) is the most extensively studied and may be more effective in HIV-infected patients who have not progressed to full-blown AIDS. Paroxetine (Paxil) is probably equally effective but has not been well studied. The major side effects for all the SSRIs include insomnia, stomach upset, transient loss of appetite, and very common sexual dysfunctions of all types.

The psychostimulants deserve a special discussion. They are probably the most effective, rapid-acting antidepressant for HIV-infected patients and are probably the first-choice medication for people with AIDS who have severe depression with extremely low energy, as well as for HIV-infected people with mild neuro-cognitive deficits like those seen in mild HIV-related dementias (Fernandez 1988). However, these medications are very addictive, can cause severe insomnia and loss of appetite, may activate a stimulant addiction in a patient in recovery, may cause paranoia and psychosis, and should be used with great caution in patients with a history of seizures.

Psychosis. With asymptomatic HIV-infected patients, psychotic symptoms are more likely to be secondary to drug intoxication (mostly cocaine or stimulants) or to a primary psychiatric disorder such as bipolar disorder or schizophrenia (Kushner 1991). In the later stages of AIDS, delirium is added to the differential diagnosis and is possibly caused by medications, infections, metabolic abnormalities, or structural CNS lesions. HIV dementia may also be associated with psychotic symptoms.

Because of the higher rates of extrapyramidal symptoms seen in HIV-infected patients, high-potency neuroleptics, such as haloperidol, should be used with caution. The best choices would be the mid-potency neuroleptics, such as thiothixine (Navane) and perphenazine (Trilafon). The low-potency neuroleptics, such as chlorpromazine (Thorazine and others), are also best avoided because of their severe anticholinergic side effects.

Providers' Attitudes

The fact that HIV-infected patients who are substance abusers are statistically more likely to "fail" in the multiple arenas of disease progression, sobriety, untreated mental illness, and other areas can have a chilling effect on their treatment. An attitude of "Why bother?" or a set of limited expectations may arise from either patients or providers. Providers may feel that the patients' drug use is a type of coping mechanism and that it would be cruel to deprive them of it when they may not have long to live. Effective treatments may be overlooked if providers assume that patients will not be able to adhere to treatment regimens. Overcoming these considerable obstacles requires much time and patience. It calls for a commitment to take the extra time to build trust with a person who has probably had many negative interactions with medical personnel. Psychiatrists and mental health professionals, including case managers, can create and support the bridges between medical care and recovery program treatment.

Primary care providers are likely to seek psychiatric consultation for the patient who presents some diagnostic confusion, who does not seem to wish to become involved in or remain consistent with his or her medical care, who seems unable to accept the HIV serostatus or the need for substance abuse intervention and treatment, or who has serious or chronic mental illness. Mental health treatment can provide the constant infusion of hope that the HIV-infected patient needs and that has been demonstrated to help in the improvement of the quality of life as well as with compliance with medical treatments.

Suicidality: A Special Concern

Suicide and HIV are inextricably linked. The psychiatric and medical literature has looked at the link between suicide and HIV infection, noting a higher incidence of suicidal ideation, suicide attempts, and actual suicide in HIV-infected patients than in the general population (Alfanso et al. 1994; Beckett and Shenson 1993). Substance abuse is an added risk factor for increased suicidal thinking and attempts, especially while a person is intoxicated. Several risk factors and information about the likelihood of suicide among patients across the entire spectrum of HIV infection (from learning one is HIV positive to having end-stage AIDS) can help the provider in making an assessment and in providing guidance (Cabaj 1994).

When providers ask about suicide, patients are usually relieved to be able to talk about feelings that they might think need to be hidden. They often take comfort in learning that suicidal thoughts are common, or even expected, in a person who is living with HIV infection.

A suicide assessment includes a complete mental status examination; a thorough history, especially of psychiatric problems or suicide attempts; a current psychosocial assessment; a review of current and past use or abuse of alcohol or other drugs; and an assessment of current medical status, including current medications. The evaluator should be more alert to suicidal ideation or intent in patients with the following:

- Current symptoms of depression
- Psychiatric history of depression, anxiety, alcohol or substance abuse, or organic mental disorders in the patient or a family member
- Experience with someone who did successfully commit a suicide that could be seen as positive or "for the best"
- History of several losses due to AIDS
- Limited or nonexistent social support system
- Inability to work and/or financial worries
- Guilt or shame over having HIV infection
- Progression in HIV illness
- Large drop in CD4 counts
- Limited future medical treatment options
- Pain that is increasing or difficult to treat
- Mild neurocognitive impairment
- Hopelessness about feeling better

The development of denial, acceptance, or even mild dementia may actually help reduce the incidence of suicidal ideation or intent in someone diagnosed with AIDS.

If the provider believes the patient is open and honest about the suicidal thinking and has no immediate plan to act on the feelings, education, support, reassurance, and the offer to be available in the future (or to provide a future referral option) usually suffice. Most patients are able to contract to refrain from acting on suicidal feelings, can promise to call someone if the suicidal intent recurs, and feel reassured that the provider is listening and taking them seriously. The option for an extra visit or increased mental health services could also be offered.

The provider may need to intervene in some way when there are factors that raise doubts about the patient's contract or that may interfere with the patient's ability to control impulsive behavior. These factors include evidence of current alcoholism, substance abuse, or a history of suicide attempts while intoxicated; severe depression; or the diagnosis of borderline personality disorder. When appropriate, the provider could counsel about reducing and stopping the substance use; consider psychotherapy for a severe depression; or refer the patient to a substance abuse counselor, provider, or program in addition to more intensive mental health interventions. In the rare instances in which a patient is clearly intending to act on suicidal feelings or cannot contract to not hurt himself or herself, the provider needs to arrange for an emergency psychiatric visit and possible admission before allowing the patient to leave the office. Enlisting the help of a lover, spouse, close friend, or family member may be a crucial and necessary step.

Psychotherapy

Although it is recognized that traditional psychotherapy, with its insight-oriented techniques, is of limited or no value with substance abusers who are actively using drugs or alcohol, psychotherapy and other mental health interventions can play a very important role in the treatment of HIV-infected substance users (Cadwell et al. 1994; Zegans et al. 1994). As noted previously, group therapy in particular may be quite helpful by allowing a focus on both the consequences of the HIV infection itself and the struggles to deal with the substance use or abuse (Tunnell 1994).

Some general themes emerge in psychotherapy with HIV-infected substance abusers who are clean and sober or are attempting to become so. These include coping with a treatable but not curable—and ultimately fatal—illness; facing the unknown and uncertainty almost daily; stigma and shame; facing ostracization; and dealing with losses and powerlessness. Although treatment options are now more hopeful for patients with AIDS and HIV infection, patients face constant media attention to treatment failures, frustrations in developing an HIV vaccine, the expense of treatment, and limited access to treatments.

Protease inhibitors have brought a new hopefulness to the treatment of HIV infection and are allowing many HIV-infected patients to return to full function, including work and socializing. Although this treatment modality is usually embraced as a positive intervention, some infected individuals have planned their lives as though they would have a short life span and are not prepared for the financial or emotional consequences of "coming back from the dead." In instances in which a protease treatment fails or is not tolerated, an HIV-infected patient can become extremely demoralized and may relapse into substance use. In addition, many uninfected people are now not as concerned about following HIV risk-reduction guidelines, under the mistaken impression that AIDS can now be cured or is only a minor inconvenience.

Even with the protease inhibitors, the HIV-infected patient faces many losses, and psychotherapy—whether individual, couples, family, or group—can be very helpful. These patients face a long list of possible losses that may be experienced as a drumroll on the way to the death chamber. Many of these patients lose their health, mobility, energy, and financial resources. They may also possibly lose sexual intimacy; the support of significant others, family, or friends; income and profession; or the hope for future relationships. Many patients report the loss of a sense of value, of the future, and of personal dignity.

Behavior change is quite difficult. Knowledge of HIV serostatus alone does not change behavior. Substance use and sex have such built-in rewards, and are so often linked, that changing these behaviors to make them less risky may be quite difficult. Psychotherapy and behavior modification can be quite useful to this end. The relapse prevention model that is often used to help substance abusers avoid picking up a drink or drug can also be used to intervene with sexually risky behavior. Patients can be taught to examine the circumstances and situation that accompanied their failure to follow risk-reduction guidelines and to apply what is learned about trigger points in future situations.

A concomitant mental health diagnosis in an HIV-infected substance abuser (so-called triple diagnosis) requires additional treatment, again with the recognition of some of the risks involved in psychopharmacology (Batki 1990b). Whether the substance abuse or the mental health condition is treated first or whether both are treated together depends on the individual patient. A psychotic, homeless, schizophrenic, HIV-infected man who is using cocaine may not benefit from most interventions unless the psychosis is treated. A depressed, HIV-infected, pregnant, African American woman who uses crack cocaine may not be able to avail herself of services until the crack use is addressed.

Special Concerns and Special Populations

Specific populations at higher risk for HIV infection may have specific psychosocial needs and issues related to their societal, cultural, or economic status. Gay and bisexual men, youth, women and children, and people of color have some unique concerns in treatment in addition to the issues noted earlier in this chapter.

Gay and Bisexual Men

Men who have sex with men (the CDC category used to report its data) may self-identify as gay (men with homosexual sexual orientation), bisexual (men who feel sexually drawn to both men and women), or heterosexual (men who have sex with men as a purely physical act and not as a reflection of an innate sexual orientation). Regardless of their sexual orientation, unprotected sexual contact will put such men at risk. Many men from minority backgrounds who have sex with other men do not self-identify as gay or bisexual. Interventions therefore need to be based not on sexual orientation but on sexual behavior.

Women who have sex with other women often also have sex with men, and certainly may use injection drugs and share needles, and so are also prone to HIV infection. Many gay men, lesbians, and bisexual people are wary of the medical establishment and may resist seeking health care, mistrust the advice given, or question the treatment plan suggested if the provider displays evidence of homophobia (the fear and hatred of gay, lesbian, and bisexual people or homosexual and bisexual sexual orientations) or heterosexism (the belief that heterosexuality is the only acceptable norm or standard) (Cabaj 1996).

To work more effectively with HIV-infected, substance-abusing, gay men, providers should understand a possible link with substance use and the formation of gay identity. For the child who will grow up to be gay, the awareness of being "different"—of having affectional and sexual longings that are different from those of others around him or her—may be evident quite early in life. Such a child hides his or her needs and longings, putting on a false front and creating a false self, because his or her true needs are often rejected or described as wrong or bad. Dissociation and denial become major defenses used to cope with internal feelings. Rejection and criticism lead to pain, denial, isolation, and fear.

Substance use serves as an easy relief that can provide acceptance and, more important, that mirrors the comforting dissociation developed in childhood. Alcohol and other drugs cause dissociation from feelings and anxiety, mimicking the emotional state that many gay people developed in childhood in order to survive. The symptom-relieving aspects of substance use help fight the effects of homophobia; they can allow "forbidden" behavior, allow social comfort in bars or other unfamiliar social settings, and provide comfort just by the dissociative state itself. Some gay people cannot imagine socializing without alcohol or other mood-altering substances. Many men had their first homosexual experiences while drinking or being drunk. This connection is a very powerful behavioral link—the pleasure and release of substance use and the pleasure and release of sex—and can be very difficult to change or unlink later in life.

The easy availability of alcohol and drugs at gay bars and parties encourages the use of substances early in the process of "coming out" and gay socialization. Substance use helps many HIV-infected gay men brace themselves for the rejection they anticipate from family, friends, or partners by coming out as a gay man, as an HIV-infected person, or both.

Because of the above factors, intervention, treatment, and recovery may be difficult for gay men, especially when HIV plays a role. Some of the suggestions and guidelines of AA and NA and most treatment programs may be more difficult for some gay men to follow. Giving up or avoiding old friends, especially fellow substance users, may be difficult when a gay person has limited contacts who relate to him as a gay person or accept him as an HIV-positive person. Staying away from bars or parties may be difficult because these are often the only social outlets. Special help on how to refrain from drinking or using drugs in such settings may therefore be necessary. The many deaths from AIDS and HIV-related conditions may weaken the support network for clean and sober gay men and lesbians and lead to the almost continuous bereavement many gay people experience.

Gay-sensitive individual and / or group psychotherapy, in addition to gay-sensitive recovery work, may be necessary for many gay patients in early recovery. Discussions about sexual orientation and awareness of the impact of HIV are absolutely necessary in detoxification and rehabilitation programs. All gay people in early recovery need help in looking at internalized homophobia and in finding ways to accept their sexual orientation.

Providers must be aware of their own personal attitudes regarding homosexuality and HIV-related conditions. If a health care provider is homophobic or fears AIDS and cannot get help in working out these attitudes with a supportive colleague or supervisor, the patient would be better off referred to another staff member for help (Cabaj 1988). Gay men with HIV infection who are facing recovery from substance abuse should not have to fight homophobia in a health care system to get quality care.

There is a growing literature on working with gay people with substance abuse (Cabaj 1996, 1997; Finnegan and McNally 1987; Gonsiorek 1985; Hart 1991; Ziebold and Mongeon 1985), as well as general literature on homosexuality, gay men, and lesbians (Cabaj and Stein 1996). There are national organizations, some with referral services, to help therapists meet the needs of their gay and lesbian patients or to help gay men and lesbians find gay-sensitive care. These include the National Association of Lesbian and Gay Addiction Professionals, the National Gay and Lesbian Health Association, the Association of Gay and Lesbian Psychiatrists, and the Gay and Lesbian Medical Association.

Youth

Society in general ignores the sexuality of youth and adolescents, and schools mostly refuse to offer objective sex education or to provide easy access to condoms. Drug use is ignored or minimized, and injection drug use is often totally denied. Youth experiment with sex with both genders and often do not understand the concept of risk because life appears to be unending and invulnerable. Using drugs is seen as defiant or as a means to cope with stress and adolescent adjustments; adults are not to be trusted.

Special sensitivity and understanding are needed to work with youth of any background, especially those who are gay or lesbian or are from an ethnic minority background. Gay male youth in particular may be subjected to harassment at home or at school and are prone to alcohol abuse, dropping out of school, running away, and getting involved in sex for drugs or money, with all the inherent risks attending these behaviors (Ku et al. 1992; Rotheram-Borus et al. 1995; Savin-Williams 1994). I have worked with many youth who—thrown out by their families for being gay, living on the streets, and using drugs—attempt to become HIV infected on purpose in order to obtain the social benefits available to people with serious HIV infections.

Women and Children

Women are still seen as being at relatively low risk for HIV infection in the United States unless they happen to use injection drugs or are the sexual partners of male IDUs or of men who have sex with men (Moscher and Pratt 1993). Outside of this country, heterosexual contact is the most frequent risk for HIV infection, and in the United States, the demographics of the HIV-infected population is changing to reflect the increased risk through heterosexual contact (CDC 1997).

Children of HIV-infected substance abusers are at risk for infection during the perinatal process, but even if uninfected, they face the sociological and economic consequences of losing a parent to AIDS (Regan-Kubinski and Sharts-Engel 1992). Children are also at risk for sexual abuse, especially in households with substance-abusing adults, and thus are at risk for HIV infection through direct sexual contact. As the age at first contact with drug use lowers in the United States, injecting drug use is not uncommon in children.

People of Color

People of color, no matter what their cultural or ethnic background, face prejudice throughout society and may well expect to encounter it in medical professionals, substance abuse programs, and social service agencies. As is true with working with gay, lesbian, and bisexual people, special sensitivity and understanding are necessary in working with minority HIV-infected substance abusers. Acceptance, openness, directness, and understanding about the limited access to treatment resources will aid in providing the most beneficial and effective medical care (Icard et al. 1992; National Commission on AIDS 1992).

Conclusions

The multiple components involved in working with HIV-infected substance abusers make mental health and substance abuse treatment challenging and exciting. Balancing cultural, ethnic, and socioeconomic factors, in addition to the consequences of stigma and prejudice in regard to sexual orientation and substance use, the provider needs to call on many skills and exercise compassion, sensitivity, and limit setting. Substance abuse does not preclude the treatment of HIV-related conditions, even with the newest and most complicated treatment regimens. In turn, having an HIV infection does not preclude intervention and treatment for coexisting substance abuse.

A recognition of both the usefulness and the limitations of psychotherapy and psychopharmacology will help the provider avoid frustrations in working with HIV-infected substance users who do not seem to respond to traditional methods. Working closely with the medical provider and allying with substance abuse treatment programs or techniques are essential for successful mental health interventions. An "all-or-nothing" mentality will prevent most substance abusers from entering treatment, and asking for total abstinence is not reasonable in most cases. Harm reduction and relapse prevention approaches are most useful.

Substance abuse treatment is HIV prevention. Working with the HIV-infected substance abuser to remain in treatment and to adhere to treatment plans, possibly with the help of intensive case management, should be combined with education about HIV risk reduction, thus helping HIV-infected patients to prevent or limit the chance of infecting others. Prevention efforts for uninfected substance abusers need to be targeted to the at-risk population, whether it be white, gay men who drink or use recreational drugs or Latino IDUs.

Providers can avoid burnout, as well as anger and frustration over substance-abusing patients who continue to use drugs or who fail to follow HIV risk-reduction guidelines when intoxicated, by recognizing the limits of the provider's role, understanding the nature of substance abuse, and acknowledging the role of the patient's responsibility. Respecting the individual patient's humanity, responsibility, and ability to make choices when judgment is not suspended while intoxicated will allow the provider to form an active partnership with the HIV-infected substance abuser and promote both direct treatment and prevention efforts.

References

Alfanso CA, Cohen MA, Aladjem AD, et al: HIV seropositivity as a major risk factor for suicide in the general hospital. Psychosomatics 35(4):368–373, 1994

American Medical Association: Draft Report of the Council on Scientific Affairs. Harm reduction: a response to Resolution 416, I-94, April 1, 1996

Baldinger S: Crystal meth's dangerous dance. OUT Magazine, December/January 1996, pp 150–155

Barthwell AG: Substance use and the puzzle of adherence. Focus: A Guide to AIDS Research and Counseling 12(9):1–4, 1997

Batki SL: Buspirone in drug users with AIDS or AIDS- related complex. J Clin Psychopharmacol 10 (suppl 3):111S–115S, 1990a

Batki SL: Drug abuse, psychiatric disorders, and AIDS: dual and triple diagnosis. West J Med 152:542–547, 1990b

Beckett A, Shenson D: Suicide risk in patients with human immunodeficiency virus infection and acquired immunodeficiency syndrome. Harvard Review of Psychiatry 1(1):27–35, 1993

Booth RE, Watters JK, Chitwood DD: HIV risk-related behaviors among injecting drug users, crack smokers, and injecting drug users who smoke crack. Am J Public Health 83:1144–1148, 1993

Brettle RP: HIV and harm reduction for injection drug users. AIDS 5:125–136, 1991

Cabaj RP: Working with male homosexual patients, I: GI problems in homosexual men. Practical Gastroenterology 9(4):7–12, 1985

Cabaj RP: Homosexuality and neurosis: considerations for psychotherapy. J Homosex 15(1–2):13–23, 1988

Cabaj RP: Assessing suicidality in the primary care setting. AIDS File 8(2):7–9, 1994

Cabaj RP: Substance abuse in gay men, lesbians, and bisexual individuals, in Textbook of Homosexuality and Mental Health. Edited by Cabaj RP, Stein TS. Washington, DC, American Psychiatric Press, 1996, pp 783–799

Cabaj RP: Gays, lesbians, and bisexuals, in Substance Abuse: A Comprehensive Textbook, 3rd Edition. Edited by Lowenson JH, Ruiz P, Millman RB, et al. Baltimore, MD, Williams & Wilkins, 1997, pp 725–733

Cabaj RP, Stein TS (eds): Textbook of Homosexuality and Mental Health. Washington, DC, American Psychiatric Press, 1996

Cadwell S, Burnham R, Forstein M (eds): Therapists on the Front Line: Psychotherapy With Gay Men in the Age of AIDS. Washington, DC, American Psychiatric Press, 1994

Calzavara LM, Coates RA, Raboud JM, et al: On-going high-risk sexual behaviors in relation to recreational drug use in sexual encounters: analysis of 5 years of data from the Toronto Sexual Contact Study. Ann Epidemiol 3:272–280, 1993

Center for Substance Abuse Treatment: Treatment for HIV-Infected Alcohol and Other Drug Abusers. Treatment Improvement Protocol No 15. Edited by Selwyn P, Batki SL. DHHS Publ No SMA 95-3038. Rockville, MD, Center for Substance Abuse Treatment, 1995

Centers for Disease Control and Prevention: HIV/AIDS surveillance report: mid-year edition. Atlanta, GA, U.S. Department of Health and Human Services, Public Health Service 9(2):8–13, 1997

Diaz RM, Ayala G: The role of substance use in the sexual lives of Latino gay men. Paper presented at the Northwest Regional Workshop on HIV Prevention Approaches for Alcohol and Drug Use Among Men Who Have Sex With Other Men. Seattle, WA, September 1997

Edlin BR, Irwin KL, Faruque S, et al: Intersecting epidemics—crack cocaine use and HIV infection among inner-city young adults. N Engl J Med 331:1422–1427, 1994

Fernandez F: Cognitive impairment due to AIDS-related complex and its response to psychostimulants. Psychosomatics 29(1):38–46, 1988

Fernandez F, Levy J: Psychopharmacology in HIV spectrum disorders. Psychiatr Clin North Am 17(1):135–148, 1994

Ferrando SJ, Wall TL, Batki SL, et al: Psychiatric morbidity, illicit drug use and adherence to AZT among injecting drug users with HIV disease. Am J Drug Alcohol Abuse 22(4):475–487, 1996

Finnegan DG, McNally EB: Dual Identities: Counseling Chemically Dependent Gay Men and Lesbians. Center City, MN, Hazelden, 1987

Gonsiorek JC (ed): A Guide to Psychotherapy With Gay and Lesbian Clients. New York, Harrington Park Press, 1985

Goode E, Troiden RR: Amyl nitrite use among homosexual men. Am J Psychiatry 136(8):1067–1069, 1979

Gorman M: Substance abuse issues in men who have sex with other men: the particular case of speed. Paper presented at the Conference on Reinventing HIV Prevention for Men Who Have Sex With Other Men, Seattle, WA, May 1994

Gorman M: Speed use and HIV transmission. Focus: A Guide to AIDS Research and Counseling 11(7):4–6, 1996

Gorman EM, Morgan P, Lambert EY: Qualitative research considerations and other issues in the study of methamphetamine use among men who have sex with other men, in Qualitative Methods in Drug Abuse and HIV Research. NIDA Research Monograph Series 157. Edited by Lambert EY, Ashery R, Needle R. Rockville, MD, National Institute on Drug Abuse, 1995, pp 156–181

Hart JE (ed): Substance Abuse Treatment: Considerations for Lesbians and Gay Men. The MART Series No 2. Boston, MA, The Mobile AIDS Resource Team, 1991

Icard LD, Schilling RF, El-Bassel N, et al: Preventing AIDS among black gay men and black gay and heterosexual male intravenous drug users. Social Work 37(5):440–445, 1992

Johnston D, Smith K, Stall R: A comparison of public health care utilization by gay men and intravenous drug users with AIDS in San Francisco. AIDS Care 6(3):303–316, 1994

Ku L, Sonenstein FL, Pleck JH: Patterns of HIV risk and prevention behavior among teenage men. Public Health Rep 107(2):131–138, 1992

Kushner SF: Substance abuse and neurological disorders, in Dual Diagnosis in Substance Abuse. Edited by Gold MS, Slaby AE. New York, Marcel Dekker, 1991, pp 75–103

Lange WR, Haetzen CA, Hickey JE: Nitrites inhalants: patterns of abuse in Baltimore and Washington, DC. Am J Drug Alcohol Abuse 14(1):29–39, 1988

Leigh BC: The relationship of substance use during sex to high risk sexual behavior. J Sex Research 27(2):199–213, 1990

Leigh BC, Stall R: Substance use and risky sexual behavior for exposure to HIV. Am Psychol 48:1035–1045, 1993

Lurie P: The Public Health Impact of Needle Exchange Programs in the United States and Abroad. Report prepared for the Centers for Disease Control and Prevention by the School of Public Health, University of California, Berkeley, and the Institute for Health Policy Studies, University of California, San Francisco. Vol I, September 1993, pp i–519; Vol II, October 1993, pp i–182; Summary, Conclusions, and Recommendations, September 1993, pp I–43

MacGregor RR: Alcohol and drugs as co-factors for AIDS, in AIDS and Substance Abuse. Edited by Siegel L. New York, Harrington Park Press, 1988, pp 47–71

Markowitz JC, Klerman GL, Clougherty KF, et al: Individual psychotherapies for depressed HIV-positive patients. Am J Psychiatry 152(10):1504–1509, 1995

Moscher WD, Pratt WF: AIDS-related behavior among women 15–44 years of age, United States, 1988 and 1990. Centers for Disease Control and Prevention Advance Data No 239, December 22, 1993

Munoz L: Positively risky: more AIDS cases feared among gay men using "sex drug" crystal meth. The Los Angeles Times, May 11, 1995

National Commission on AIDS: The Challenge of HIV/AIDS in Communities of Color. Washington, DC, National Commission on AIDS, 1992

Nix C, Cabaj RP: Case management for HIV-infected substance abusers. Focus: A Guide to AIDS Research and Counseling 7(10):5–6, 1992

Novick DM, Joseph H: Medical maintenance: the treatment of chronic opiate dependence in general medical practice. J Subst Abuse Treat 8:233–239, 1991

Nyamathi A, Flaskerud J, Leake B, et al: Impoverished women at risk for AIDS: social support variables. J Psychosoc Nurs Ment Health Serv 34(11):31–39, 1996

Ostrow DG: Substance abuse and HIV infection. Psychiatr Clin North Am 17(1):69–89, 1994

Ostrow DG: Substance use, HIV, and gay men. Focus: A Guide to AIDS Research and Counseling 11(7):1–3, 1996

Ostrow DG: The science and politics of interventions for alcohol and drug abusing men who have sex with men: a review and commentary on progress since 1986. Paper presented at the Northwest Regional Workshop on HIV Prevention Approaches for Alcohol and Drug Use Among Men Who Have Sex With Other Men, Seattle, WA, September 1997

Ostrow DG, McKirnan D: Prevention of substance-related high-risk sexual behavior among gay men: critical review of the literature and proposed harm reduction approaches. Journal of the Gay and Lesbian Medical Association 1(2):97–110, 1997

Paul JP, Stall RD, Crosby GM, et al: Correlates of sexual risk-taking among gay male substance abusers. Addiction 89:971–983, 1994

Perkins DO, Leserman J, Stern RA, et al: Somatic symptoms and HIV infection: relationship of depressive symptoms and indicators of HIV disease. Am J Psychiatry 152(12):1776–1781, 1995

Rabkin JG, Rabkin R, Harrison W, et al: Effect of imipramine on mood and enumerative measures of immune status in depressed patients with HIV illness. Am J Psychiatry 151(4):516–523, 1994a

Rabkin JG, Wagner G, Rabkin R: Effects of sertraline on mood and immune status in patients with major depression and HIV illness: an open trial. J Clin Psychiatry 55(10):433–439, 1994b

Regan-Kubinski MJ, Sharts-Engel N: The HIV-infected woman: illness cognition assessment. Journal of Psychosocial Nursing 30(2):11–15, 1992

Rotheram-Borus MJ, Rosario M, Reid H, et al: Predicting patterns of sexual acts among homosexual and bisexual youth. Am J Psychiatry 152(4):588–595, 1995

Sadownick: Kneeling at the crystal cathedral: the alarming new epidemic of methamphetamine abuse in the gay community. Genre Magazine, January 1994, pp 34–38

San Francisco Chronicle: Study shows flaws of new AIDS drugs. The San Francisco Chronicle, September 30, 1997a, pp A1, A10

San Francisco Chronicle: Even addicts can stick with AIDS drugs. The San Francisco Chronicle, October 8, 1997b, p A6

Savin-Williams RC: Verbal and physical abuse as stressors in the lives of lesbian, gay male, and bisexual youths: association with school problems, running away, substance abuse, prostitution, and suicide. J Consult Clin Psychol 62(2):261–269, 1994

Selwyn PA: Primary care for patients with human immunodeficiency virus (HIV) infection in a methadone maintenance treatment program. Ann Intern Med 111:761–763, 1989

Shoptaw S, Frosch D: Substance abuse treatment as HIV prevention for men who have sex with men. Paper presented at the Northwest Regional Workshop on HIV Prevention Approaches for Alcohol and Drug Use Among Men Who Have Sex With Other Men, Seattle, WA, September 1997

Sorenson JL, Batki SL: Management of the psychosocial sequelae of HIV infection among drug abusers, in Substance Abuse: A Comprehensive Textbook, 2nd Edition. Edited by Lowinson JK, Ruiz P, Millman RB, et al. Baltimore, MD, Williams & Wilkins, 1992, pp 788–792

Springer E: Effective AIDS prevention with active drug users: the harm reduction model. Journal of Chemical Dependency Treatment 4(2):141–157, 1991

Stall R: The prevention of HIV infection associated with drug and alcohol use during sexual activity, in AIDS and Substance Abuse. Edited by Siegel L. New York, Harrington Park Press, 1988, pp 73–88

Stall R: Intertwining epidemics: a review of research on non-intravenous substance use and abuse among gay men and their relationships to the AIDS epidemic. Paper presented at the Northwest Regional Workshop on HIV Prevention Approaches for Alcohol and Drug Use Among Men Who Have Sex With Other Men, Seattle, WA, September 1997

Stall R, McKusick L, Wiley J: Alcohol and drug use during sexual activity and compliance with safe sex guidelines for AIDS: The AIDS Behavior Research Project. Health Educ Q 13:359–371, 1986

Strang J: Harm reduction for drug users: exploring the dimensions of harm, their measurement, and strategies for reductions. AIDS and Public Policy Journal 7(3):145–152, 1992

Tunnell G: Special issues in group psychotherapy for gay men with AIDS, in Therapists on the Front Line: Psychotherapy With Gay Men in the Age of AIDS. Edited by Cadwell S, Burnham R, Forstein M. Washington, DC, American Psychiatric Press, 1994, pp 237–254

Wall TL: Adherence to zidovudine (AZT) among HIV-infected methadone patients: a pilot study of supervised therapy and dispensing compared to usual care. Drug Alcohol Depend 37:261–269, 1995

White JC: HIV risk assessment and prevention in lesbians and women who have sex with women: practical information for clinicians. Health Care for Women International 18(2):127–138, 1997

Zegans LS, Gerhard AL, Coates TJ: Psychotherapies for the person with HIV disease. Psychiatr Clin North Am 17(1):149–162, 1994

Ziebold TO, Mongeon JE (eds): Gay and Sober: Directions for Counseling and Therapy. New York, Harrington Park Press, 1985

Chapter 5

Contemporary Issues in Dual Diagnosis

H. Westley Clark, M.D., J.D., M.P.H., and
Terry Michael McClanahan, M.A.

The principles and practice of contemporary psychiatry require an understanding that any patient who presents with a psychological complaint may also be using alcohol or psychoactive drugs, licit or illicit—either of which complicate the presenting picture. Because the use of substances of abuse is widespread, it is critical for the evaluating or treating psychiatrist to be aware of the complexities created by a presenting symptom in a person who also uses alcohol or drugs. The term *dual diagnosis* is one of convenience used to capture the concept that some patients may have a substance use disorder in addition to another psychiatric disorder.

Inherent in the concept of dual diagnosis is the task of differentiating the effects of the psychoactive substance(s) from the symptoms of the other psychiatric disorder. Hence the question would become, for example, whether the auditory hallucinations of a person with schizophrenia are due to the schizophrenia or to the methamphetamine that the person is injecting.

In the public sector, *dual diagnosis* has been a useful term to address the provision of services to those patients who require services from a mental health clinic and from a drug or alcohol treatment clinic. Dually diagnosed patients have also become symbols for programmatic inefficiencies—the duplication of services, the denial of services, or the failure to provide services to patients presenting to a mental health clinic that is forbidden to treat alcohol or drug abusers or who present to a substance abuse

This chapter was supported in part by Grant 1P50-DA09253 from the National Institute on Drug Abuse (Sharon Hall, Principal Investigator).

clinic that is forbidden to treat psychiatric disorders other than substance abuse.

In this chapter, we discuss a spectrum of issues inherent in the concept of dual diagnosis. We describe assessment strategies that can help the practicing clinician to differentiate probable primary substance abuse problems from psychiatric disorders other than substance abuse. We address issues of psychopharmacology, which is an important area of concern for the practicing physician. Finally, we summarize some of the psychosocial issues that are fundamental in the treatment process for dual diagnosis.

Epidemiology

The results from the Epidemiologic Catchment Area (ECA) study are still frequently cited in estimates of the prevalence of specific disorders in the United States. Although the reported data in the ECA on the comorbidity of mental disorders and substance abuse are more than a decade old, they still capture the magnitude of the problem of these co-occurring conditions.

The specific substance abuse problems detailed in the ECA include abuse of or dependence on alcohol, marijuana, cocaine, opiates, barbiturates, amphetamines, and hallucinogens. The specific mental disorders include schizophrenia, antisocial personality disorder, anxiety disorders, and affective (mood) disorders. Comorbidity is detailed using the non–substance abuse disorder as the anchor and using the substance abuse disorder as the anchor. The usefulness of this characterization depends on the clinical site at which the patient presents. In a dichotomized health care system, a patient with comorbid disorders who is identified as having one type of problem as primary may have the other type of problem ignored.

The ECA (Regier et al. 1990) data indicated that 47% of all individuals with a lifetime diagnosis of schizophrenia or schizophreniform disorders have met the criteria for substance abuse or dependence. Furthermore, the odds of having a diagnosis of substance abuse are almost five times as high for patients with schizophrenia than for the general population.

The ECA data indicated that 23.7% of individuals with an anxiety disorder also have a substance abuse disorder. More specifically, however, of those patients with panic disorder, 35.8% also have a substance use disorder. Of those with obsessive-compulsive disorder, some 32.8% also have a substance use disorder.

A substance use disorder is found in 32.0% of patients with an affective disorder, according to the ECA data. Overall, the rates of alcohol abuse or dependence are nearly equal to those of other drug abuse in patients with an affective disorder. Within the affective disorders, the prevalence of substance use disorders is 60.7% among those individuals with bipolar I disorder.

The basic prevalence rates of the ECA data will naturally be altered depending on the specific populations being addressed in a given situation and the methods used to assess the epidemiology of a specific phenomenon. Hence, patients presenting in the psychiatric emergency department may demonstrate one pattern, whereas those presenting in an outpatient clinic may manifest another pattern. In one report, for instance, Claassen et al. (1997) found that clinicians' suspicions of drug use among psychotic patients in the emergency department lacked specificity because potential use was suspected by clinicians in a large number of cases in which toxicology screens were negative.

In a recent report on the psychiatric and substance use comorbidity among 716 men and women seeking opioid outpatient methadone treatment, Brooner et al. (1997) determined that 47% had a lifetime psychiatric diagnosis. Furthermore, the gender differentiation revealed an almost equal distribution between males and females (48% versus 47%, respectively).

Brooner et al. (1997) reported that among a sample of opioid abusers with Axis I disorders alone, mood disorders (19%) and anxiety disorders (8.2%) predominated among lifetime diagnoses, and schizophrenia occurred at a much lower level (0.1%). These disorders showed a difference in rates based on gender. Among females, the lifetime prevalence of mood disorder was 27.5% (11.4% in men), that of anxiety disorders was 10.7% (6.1% in men), and that of schizophrenia was 0.3% (0.0% in men). Thus, although 24% of the sample may have had a lifetime prevalence of any Axis I disorder, females (33.4%) were twice as likely as males (15.6%) to have an Axis I disorder.

The question of whether an Axis I diagnosis was induced by

substance abuse or was independent in the treatment-seeking opioid users was also addressed in this report. It was concluded that major depression was most often substance induced (78% of the affected sample), whereas in half of the subjects with dysthymic disorder and one-fifth of those with panic disorder, the disorder was considered to be substance induced.

Among patients with Axis II disorders assessed in the report of Brooner et al. (1997), male opioid users presenting for treatment were more likely to have a personality disorder (40.5%) than were women (28.4%). Males were more likely than females to have antisocial personality (33.9% and 15.4%, respectively) and paranoid personality (4.5% and 1.8%, respectively). However, females were more likely than males to be diagnosed with borderline personality disorder (9.5% versus 1.3%), avoidant personality (7.1% versus 3.4%), dependent personality (3.0% versus 0.5%), and histrionic personality (2.1% versus 0.8%).

Brooner et al. (1997) also looked at the lifetime and current rates of substance use disorders in their population of opioid-dependent patients who presented for treatment. Although dependence on cocaine (64.7%), cannabis (50.8%), alcohol (50.3%), and sedatives (44.6%) was quite common in this population in terms of lifetime rates, only dependence on cocaine (40.2%) and alcohol (24.7%) demonstrated a current rate of greater than 20%.

In summary, the report of Brooner et al. (1997) has epidemiological importance because of the reviewed psychiatric findings of a large sample of substance users who presented for opioid treatment. Multiple demographic variables were reviewed, including gender, age, education, and minority status. This study clearly built on the ECA data, as the authors compared some of their findings with the ECA data. Finally, by presenting a more contemporary analysis, the authors were able to conclude that methadone maintenance alone would not address the needs of the patient population served and that specialized interventions would be necessary to effect substantial changes in the outcome.

Basic Assessment, Evaluation, and Diagnosis

The fundamental issue in diagnosing a patient who presents with a comorbid condition is differentiating the disorders. For instance, approximately 111 million Americans are current consumers of alcohol (National Institute on Drug Abuse 1996); that is, they have consumed at least one drink within the past month. This statistic, however, can be misleading. The problem becomes more apparent when one examines the number of heavy drinkers (defined as those who have had five or more drinks on five or more occasions within the past month), of which there are approximately 32 million in the United States. When that figure is confounded with the approximately 45 million Americans with a psychiatric disorder, the complexity of the issue becomes apparent. The traditional approach to assessment, diagnosis, and treatment has been to consider the two disorders as separate diagnoses with separate treatments.

Assessment and diagnosis are pivotal components in the treatment of dually diagnosed patients. Assessing the mental health patient for substance abuse is even more vital in the light of findings that the prevalence of substance abuse among this population is estimated to range from one-third to one-half (Carey et al. 1996). Goldfinger et al. (1996) reported a similar finding—that two-thirds of their subjects were diagnosed as having a lifetime substance abuse disorder. Boyd and Hauenstein (1997) reported that the prevalence of comorbid disorders in substance-abusing populations ranges from as low as 3% to as high as 98%. In their research with dual disorders in rural substance-abusing females, Boyd and Hauenstein (1997) found a prevalence rate of 63.3% in their female subjects.

Traditional assessment begins with a clinical interview, in which the clinician takes a thorough history. Guiding the clinician during this process is a knowledge of DSM-IV (American Psychiatric Association 1994). Although DSM-IV is theoretically only a guide, it is the standard from which clinicians operate. Clinical judgment allows the clinician to deviate and to assess the clinical significance of any one criterion. As Hasin et al. (1996) indicate, the differentiation between organic and nonorganic disease is left up to the clinician.

Research has firmly established the existence of certain clusters of comorbidity. For instance, the prevalence of antisocial personality disorder is elevated in male opioid abusers, and that of borderline personality disorder is elevated among women who abuse alcohol and drugs. There are two traditional schools of thought in regard to dual diagnosis. The first is that the psychiatric condition is primary and that when it is treated effectively, the substance abuse problem will consequently diminish. The second school of thought is that the substance abuse is of primary concern and that once that condition is treated effectively, the psychiatric condition will consequently diminish in acuity and chronicity. Helzer and Pryzbeck (1988) found that a comorbid psychiatric diagnosis is present among 44% of male alcoholic patients and 65% of female alcoholic patients. Furthermore, they also reported that the most common comorbid psychiatric diagnosis in these females was major depressive disorder.

The problem with most assessment instruments in mental health settings is that they rely upon self-report. This is problematic in that substance abuse within this setting is underreported (Carey 1996). These findings indicate the importance of the need to use valid instruments for patients who present to the psychiatric setting. Also embedded within this statement is the issue of the reliability of self-report.

Goldfinger et al. (1996) also report that nondisclosure is a significant problem in the assessment of homeless mentally ill persons. When data are gathered from multiple sources, corroborating evidence is essential for an accurate diagnosis. As Goldfinger et al. (1996) reported, most single-method approaches to identifying substance abuse among mentally ill persons are inadequate. Collateral data can be gained from various members of the treatment team, family members, or multiple assessment instruments, including behavioral charting of the substance use. Goldfinger et al. (1996) found three clusters in regard to dual diagnosis: moderate dual diagnostic problems, a multiproblem cluster, and a cluster characterized by distress over psychiatric, family, and employment problems.

The instruments most widely used and accepted as measures of substance abuse are the Structured Clinical Interview using the DSM-IV (SCID) (Spitzer et al. 1990), the Addiction Severity Index (ASI) (McClellan et al. 1992), and the Symptom Checklist (SCL-90-R) (Derogatis 1983). The SCID has long been used in the psychiatric setting to diagnose and determine the severity of substance use and abuse. The drug and alcohol section of the ASI gathers data for evaluating the history of substance use, treatment, and frequency of use within the past month. The SCID also assesses current usage as well as lifetime history.

Reliability data have been reported for the ASI in both substance-related and psychiatric disorders (Hodgins and El-Guebaly 1992). Appleby et al. (1997) report strong correlations between the SCID—Patient Version (SCID-P) and the ASI. However, in the area of dual diagnosis, the ASI is inadequate in assessing whether the psychological symptoms are primary or secondary. The SCL-90-R is most often used to obtain information regarding current use and psychological distress.

Contemporary Assessment and Legal Implications

Our position in regard to dually diagnosed individuals is that substance abuse is a psychiatric disorder that cannot and should not be separated from other psychiatric conditions. Accordingly, its treatment cannot and should not be segregated from that of a concurrent psychiatric condition.

Substance abuse may arise from either interpersonal or intrapersonal issues and is a coping mechanism to help ameliorate additional psychiatric symptoms (Janssen 1994). From a self psychology perspective, when one is unable to soothe oneself in times of stress, the soothing may come from a bottle, a needle, a pipe, or a line. Therefore, a key issue in the assessment of substance use and abuse within this context is that any assessment instrument must be complemented with an in-depth clinical interview.

Clinicians should also be aware of the fact that severe psychiatric patients are still protected under the Fifth and Fourteenth Amendments, in which the underlying principle of liberty is protected by due process. Due process has two components: procedural due process and substantive due process. Under procedural due process, the state must provide notice to the individual in such a way as to allow him or her the opportunity to be heard in a fair and impartial manner. Individuals who are dually diagnosed are protected against civil commitment unless the situation is an emergency. Not withstanding emergency proceedings, a civil commitment requires the state to conduct an impartial hearing before it can involuntarily hospitalize an individual under psychiatric conditions (Bersoff et al. 1994). *Zinermon v. Burch* (1990) requires that professionals act sensitively to the treatment needs of their patients as well as to their rights to procedural due process.

Under substantive due process, the state must ensure that the individual's constitutional rights are protected. For instance, even under a very rigorous procedural due process hearing, the evidence must be based on sound judgment and rationale. Within this context, it is quite evident that clinical judgments should whenever possible be supported by psychometrically tested instruments that can both aid in the treatment of the presenting patient and provide guidance for treatment.

Bersoff et al. (1994) offer the following advice for the psychiatric professional concerning the assessment and treatment of persons with dual diagnoses:

- It is important to understand the ethical constraints on professional behavior.
- Advocacy, protection, and representation of dual diagnoses require a heightened understanding of this population and their rights, because these individuals may have difficulties in comprehending the legal mechanisms that are available for their protection.
- The professional has an obligation to respect the patient's self-determination and autonomy interests as well as his or her due process rights.
- Practitioners should use psychometrically sound instruments.
- The duty of fidelity belongs to the patient, not the institution, the legal system, or the public.

A major reason for this discussion of legal issues is that patients with comorbid conditions may be deprived of state-sanctioned benefits if it is determined that their primary problem is substance abuse rather than, for example, schizophrenia or bipolar affective disorder (BAD). Social Security benefits, Veterans Affairs benefits, worker's compensation benefits, or other social welfare benefits may hinge on the accurate assessment of the presenting problems. Even public housing benefits can be denied to a patient with a primary diagnosis of substance abuse. A hasty conclusion that the patient's primary diagnosis is alcoholism or cocaine dependence may result in the denial or termination of social welfare benefits.

Consequently, the risks associated with diagnosis and assessment are not restricted to the use of a medication that is not indicated or the employment of a treatment that is inappropriate. Thus, the patient bears the risks of misdiagnosis, whether it is direct, in the form of inappropriate treatment, or indirect, in the form of denial of social benefits.

Psychopharmacotherapeutics

When a psychiatric patient presents for general treatment, the treating physician must determine whether the presenting symptoms are secondary to substance abuse or are directly related to a psychiatric disorder other than substance use. Unlike psychiatric patients in general, dually diagnosed patients present with a history of both substance use–related and non-substance use–related psychiatric disorders. Thus, the treating psychiatrist may at any one time be treating the sequelae of substance abuse, the non-substance use–related psychiatric condition, or a combination of both.

This complexity demands the careful attention of the treating physician. The problem, however, has been that reliable research data have not been readily available. Unfortunately, the published literature remains woefully inadequate in informing the practicing clinician. Nevertheless, clinical strategies that provide novel approaches to treating dually diagnosed patients have been empirically formulated (Pechter et al. 1997).

The major non–substance use psychiatric disorders, such as schizophrenia, depression, and anxiety disorders, are often treated with medications. The development of pharmacotherapies for primary substance abuse disorders has not paralleled the progress apparent in the treatment of non–substance use psychiatric disorders. However, progress has been made in our clinical understanding of the treatment of both substance abuse disorders and the psychiatric sequelae of substance abuse disorders in dually diagnosed patients.

Some argue that "a patient who is actively using alcohol or drugs represents an unstable platform on which to build pharmacotherapeutic homeostasis" (Gastfriend 1997, p. 486). Although it is preferable to pharmacologically address the non–substance use psychiatric disorder without the disruption of the pharmacodynamic and pharmacokinetic states produced by alcohol and other drugs, the treating physician may not have the luxury of waiting very long. Thus, if the patient is known by the system providing care, the physician is able to operate with the patient's history in mind.

The treating physician may be confronted by a spectrum of clinical symptoms that may include delirium, amnestic disorder or dementia, psychosis, mood disorder, anxiety disorder, or sleep disorder. These symptoms may be produced during states of intoxication or withdrawal from stimulants (e.g., amphetamines and cocaine), hallucinogens and phencyclidine, alcohol, opioids, or sedatives. When these symptoms occur in a patient with no history of psychiatric pathology other than substance use, the clinician must determine whether psychopharmacology is indicated. This assessment is usually made with the view that, in the absence of pronounced psychosocial dysfunction caused by the substance-related clinical state, no psychopharmacology is preferred. In other words, no drugs should be used when no drugs are indicated.

The use of drugs of abuse by patients with other psychiatric conditions continues to be enigmatic. However, the locus of the reinforcing effects of a number of drugs of abuse is thought to be in the mesocorticolimbic dopamine system and its related connections.

Neurobiological findings indicate that alcoholism and drug addiction are related to abnormalities in serotonin, dopamine, and other centrally acting neurotransmitters. Depression, anxiety, and obsessive-compulsive disorders have been associated with disturbances in the endogenous serotonin system. Furthermore, serotonin has been implicated in alcohol consumption: Enhanced serotonin transmission decreases alcohol consumption, whereas serotonin depletion facilitates alcohol consumption.

The role of serotonin in stimulant abuse is less clear. However, there are indications that serotonin may play a role in the modulation of cocaine craving (Buydens-Branchey et al. 1997). Furthermore, some of amphetamine's behavioral effects may be modified by serotonin (Grady et al. 1996).

Dopamine has been implicated in both alcohol and drug abuse. In addition, in patients with schizophrenia, dopamine is associated with a heightened state of arousal that has little to do with pleasure. Furthermore, attention-deficit disorder is linked to abnormal dopamine transmission.

The choice of medications for the treatment of patients with both substance abuse disorders and Axis I non–substance abuse disorders continues to be determined on an empirical basis. Nevertheless, some advances are being made in pharmacotherapy studies of substance use and specific disorders, such as depression and schizophrenia. There is also progress in the treatment of the specific disorders themselves. Research in the neurosciences is also opening the door to novel approaches to pharmacotherapy treatments.

The key issue in the pharmacological treatment of dual psychiatric disorders is the principle that at least two conditions may require treatment. For example, the selection of a medication that appears to benefit an anxiety disorder, such as lorazepam, may exacerbate a co-occurring substance use disorder, such as alcoholism. Alternatively, the use of carbamazepine as a mood stabilizer in a patient who is also on methadone maintenance may produce withdrawal as a result of the increased metabolism of the methadone caused by the carbamazepine.

Medication Noncompliance

Prior to discussing specific medications and specific psychiatric diagnoses associated with dual diagnosis, it is important to note that medication noncompliance is a frequently observed phenomenon among dually diagnosed patients. Current substance abuse is strongly associated with medication noncompliance (Owen et al. 1996). Medication noncompliance is also associated with poor symptom outcomes. Interventions designed to decrease substance use should also incorporate efforts to decrease medication noncompliance.

Neuroleptics

For patients with psychotic disorders, the use of neuroleptics is common and not unexpected. However, the use of the neuroleptic medication creates a unique situation. The side effects of the neuroleptic medication may be problematic for patients. As a result, patients may self-medicate with the use of nonprescribed psychoactive agents to manage the negative side effects of the medications.

The traditional, or "typical," neuroleptic agents have significant central nervous system effects, including extrapyramidal symptoms, tardive dyskinesia, sedation, and dulling of cognition. Other significant side effects include neuroleptic malignant syndrome, orthostatic hypotension, liver function abnormalities, antiadrenergic and anticholinergic effects, and sexual dysfunction (Casey 1997). Although clozapine represents the advent of the "atypical" neuroleptics, it requires clinical monitoring for cardiovascular, neurological, and hematological adverse effects. The newer atypical neuroleptics have a more favorable profile of side effects, the most common of which are weight gain and changes in liver function tests and blood pressure. Furthermore, the atypical neuroleptics are as effective as the typical neuroleptics in treating the positive symptoms of schizophrenia but are more effective for the treatment of the negative symptoms.

In patients with schizophrenia, self-medication behavior is also thought to apply to both the negative and the positive symptoms of the disease. However, some contend that the self-medication hypothesis is an insufficient explanation for the concomitant use of drugs or the abusive use of alcohol in dually diagnosed patients. Despite the absence of rigorous data, it appears that many clinicians and patients endorse the notion of self-medication. Fortunately, newer neuroleptics, such as clozapine, risperidone, and olanzapine, may aid in answering the question about self-medication because they have a different side effect profile from that of traditional neuroleptics.

Wilkins (1997) noted that pharmacotherapy for patients with schizophrenia who are using cocaine may be augmented by the additional use of desipramine. In one case study, the use of clozapine, an atypical antipsychotic agent with antagonism for 5-hydroxytryptamine (serotonin); high affinity for dopamine, subtype 4 (D_4), receptor; and sparing of some dopaminergic pathways, resulted in the clinical improvement of a man with schizoaffective disorder, bipolar type, and cocaine abuse (Yovell 1994). The patient in this case had a long-term history of frequent exacerbations, multiple hospitalizations, and trials of many neuroleptics. Medication noncompliance and cocaine abuse marked this patient's clinical course. However, after the addition of clozapine to his medical regimen, the patient was compliant and free of cocaine use over a 14-month follow-up period.

A report from a community mental health center (Marcus and Snyder 1995) described some 13 patients with histories of substance abuse and schizophrenia who were treated with clozapine. All 13 of the patients had histories of nicotine dependence; 8 had histories of other substance abuse, including abuse of alcohol (n = 6), marijuana (n = 6), cocaine (n = 2), heroin (n = 1), and hallucinogens (n = 2). Of the 13 patients, 11 reported reduced use or complete abstinence after taking clozapine.

Others believe that clozapine's D_1 blocking activity and minimal D_2 blocking gives it great promise for use in patients with schizophrenia and substance use disorders. The D_1 receptor may very well be the primary receptor for the reinforcement of abuse of cocaine and other substances (Self et al. 1996).

Flupentixol, a thioxanthene derivative that effects D_2 pre- and postsynaptic receptor blockade, has been reported to produce positive results in an open-label trial of eight patients with schizophrenia who were abusing cocaine (Wilkins 1997). Decreases were observed in cocaine-positive urinalyses and in negative symptoms, suggesting the need for a more rigorous trial of this medication for the comorbid condition of schizophrenia and cocaine abuse.

Berger et al. (1996), in a study on cocaine cue-induced craving, reported that exposure to cocaine cues produced significant increases in levels of cortisol, homovanillic acid (HVA), and adrenocorticotropic hormone (ACTH) and in anxiety. Craving and anxiety were antagonized by pretreatment with haloperidol. Thus, one would suppose that the use of dopamine antagonists such as haloperidol would result in reductions in cocaine or methamphetamine use. However, it is believed that the side effect profile of haloperidol and similar drugs mitigates against their ability to reduce cocaine craving.

Mood Stabilizers

Bipolar affective episodes. BAD is clearly associated with a high risk for concomitant drug or alcohol abuse. The National Institute of Mental Health ECA study revealed that 56.1% of individuals with any bipolar disorder also had a lifetime prevalence of alcohol or drug abuse (Regier et al. 1990). Sonne et al. (1994) studied a population of individuals with BAD and found that individuals with both BAD and substance use disorder (SUD) had an earlier onset of the mood disorder, were almost four times more likely to have still other Axis I disorders, and had more hospitalizations for current substance use than did individuals without substance use disorders.

K. T. Brady et al. (1995) pointed out that, despite the high prevalence of substance abuse and dependence among patients with bipolar disorder, little information is available about the pharmacological treatment of patients with both conditions. The decision to use pharmacological agents in patients with both BAD and substance use disorders must occur within the context of differentiating, where possible, the contribution of substances like amphetamines, cocaine, or steroids. There does appear to be an association between the type of BAD and substance abuse. Patients with mixed and rapid-cycling BAD tend to have more associated alcoholism than those with less complex BAD (Keller et al. 1986).

One small, open-label, nonblinded study of nine patients with manic or mixed manic episodes and substance use disorders found that valproate appears to be safe and efficacious in the acute treatment of patients with both BAD and substance use disorders (K. T. Brady et al. 1995). It should be noted that this study found a slight elevation in liver enzymes in four of the nine patients; no patient had an elevation of greater than two times normal. Finally, the study found that the number of days of self-reported substance use was lower during the period of medication use than during the period before medication use. Although the authors did not claim a cause-and-effect relationship between valproate use and substance use, it is important to recognize that the subjects did experience an acute remission of mania as well as a decrease in substance use.

Although not specific to patients with BAD, a 12-week, randomized, double-blind, placebo-controlled, fixed-dose, outpatient study (Halikas et al. 1997) reported that, compared with placebo, carbamazepine produced a decrease in the rate of positive cocaine urinalyses and a reduction in the intensity and duration of craving. In that study, it appeared that 400 mg of carbamazepine produced better results than did 800 mg. It was also noted that higher serum levels of carbamazepine were associated with a lower rate of cocaine-positive urinalyses, fewer days of self-reported cocaine use, and briefer craving episodes. Because carbamazepine is an effective mood stabilizer for BAD, careful scrutiny is warranted for patients who have both BAD and cocaine dependence and are being treated with carbamazepine. Replication of the data of Halikas et al. (1997) in a study population with BAD would be quite encouraging. Alternatively, if carbamazepine does not produce the same effects in a study population with BAD and substance use disorders, this would also be intriguing.

Although lithium is still considered to be the drug of choice for the treatment of manic episodes, its role in the treatment of substance abuse is limited. The best function of this medication would probably be the stabilization of the patient's manic state in order to permit engagement in treatment. For dually diagnosed patients, being in any kind of treatment offers the clinician an opportunity to intervene in the substance abuse issues. In short, lithium is not currently viewed as beneficial in treating primary substance abuse problems.

Major depression. As previously mentioned, it is quite common for those using alcohol or other drugs to experience depressive symptoms at some point. Clinicians must determine whether the depressive symptoms are transient—associated with ongoing or discontinued use of a particular psychoactive substance, such as alcohol, cocaine, or heroin—or sustained, in which case they require some kind of medication. If a patient with depressive symptoms is treated with medications prematurely and inappropriately, then the patient may have to experience unnecessary side effects from the medication for an undetermined amount of time. Nevertheless, the clinician may decide that treatment with an antidepressant is warranted.

The serotonin-specific reuptake inhibitors (SSRIs) are preferred for the treatment of depressive symptoms in patients with alcoholism or drug addiction. The SSRIs themselves may have some marginal effect in reducing the consumption of alcohol (Gorelick and Paredes 1992) and cocaine (O'Brien 1996). However, it should be noted that several placebo-controlled trials have found fluoxetine to be ineffective for the treatment of cocaine dependence (Grabowsky et al. 1995). The side effect profile of the SSRIs make them the preferred drugs of choice for the treatment of depression.

Kranzler et al. (1996) found that, in the absence of a concomitant mood or anxiety disorder, type B alcoholic subjects—individuals with high levels of premorbid vulnerability, impulsivity, and alcohol-related problems—had poorer drinking-related outcomes with fluoxetine than with placebo treatment. In fact, these authors recommended that, in the absence of a comorbid mood or anxiety disorder, fluoxetine should not be used to maintain abstinence or to reduce drinking in type B alcoholic patients. In order to provide clinically useful treatment, the clinician should have some idea of whether a patient is a type A (low-risk, low-severity) or a type B (high-risk, high-severity) alcoholic.

The older, tricyclic antidepressants have been used to treat depression as well as alcoholism and other substance abuse. Although data clearly indicate that tricyclic antidepressants are effective in the treatment of depression, they are less impressive when depression is concomitant with the use of alcohol or other drugs. Still, studies continue to be conducted that suggest an effective role for the tricyclic antidepressants in the treatment of depression among alcoholic patients (Mason et al. 1996; McGrath et al. 1996). Some data suggest that imipramine is effective for alcoholism with comorbid depression (Nunes et al. 1993).

Although desipramine may be of limited usefulness in cocaine-using patients without comorbid depression, data suggest that positive results may occur for cocaine-using patients with depression. Thus, desipramine may facilitate normalization of mood, reduction of cocaine craving and use, and enhancement of treatment participation and retention (Ziedonis and Kosten 1991).

Anxiety disorders. Similar to the transient nature of depression related to substance use, concomitant anxiety symptoms may actually be secondary to substance use or withdrawal. Patients with secondary anxiety may have generalized anxiety, panic attacks, or agoraphobia for up to 6 months before experiencing spontaneous remission. However, the use of stimulants, hallucinogens, alcohol, marijuana, and other drugs may result in the onset of a sustained anxiety disorder that does not remit spontaneously (Castaneda et al. 1996). Finally, many patients with anxiety disorders are convinced that their substance use is secondary to a primary anxiety disorder. Posttraumatic stress disorder (PTSD) is an anxiety disorder that is often associated with substance use and is not etiologically secondary to substance use or withdrawal syndromes.

When the use of a pharmacological agent is deemed to be warranted in a particular patient, the choice of medication should be made from among the SSRIs, the tricyclic antidepressants, and buspirone. Benzodiazepines as a class should be avoided in patients with primary or true comorbid anxiety disorders. Mueller et al. (1996) prospectively studied 343 subjects in an anxiety disorders clinic. One group had histories of anxiety and alcohol use or dependence, whereas another had a history of anxiety without alcohol use. Over a 12-month follow-up period, the authors found that a history of an alcohol use disorder was not a strong predictor of benzodiazepine abuse in subjects with anxiety disorders.

The SSRIs, such as fluoxetine, fluvoxamine, paroxetine, and

sertraline, should be considered the drugs of choice for symptoms of PTSD, panic, and compulsions. Furthermore, trazodone may be useful for both anxiety and insomnia associated with anxiety disorders such as PTSD. Clinically, trazodone works quite well in patients with anxiety who either are decreasing or are free of substance use.

Like the SSRIs, the tricyclic antidepressants have been demonstrated to reduce anxiety symptoms in patients with both anxiety and substance use disorders. Also like the SSRIs, however, the tricyclics have only a marginal ability to decrease any concurrent substance abuse. In patients with coexisting anxiety and substance abuse, the clinician should expect pharmacotherapy to have the greatest impact on the anxiety symptoms. Thus, to the extent that the substance use is secondary to the anxiety, a reduction in substance use would follow.

Buspirone may also produce relief in patients with substance use disorders and anxiety (Kranzler et al. 1994). Patients receiving buspirone should be educated about the slower onset of action of benzodiazepines and the absence of the "high" or "rush" that may be associated with their use. In addition to patient education about the effects of the drug, it is critical to provide support for the patient in tolerating the slow and delayed period of effect, which may be as long as 6 weeks.

The long-term use of therapeutic doses of benzodiazepines can produce symptoms of physiological dependence in as many as 100% of patients. For this reason, it is clear that care must be exercised in prescribing such agents to patients with anxiety who have comorbid substance abuse histories. It is also well known that most benzodiazepines can induce nontherapeutic use in many patients. Even the longer-acting, slow-onset benzodiazepines, such as clonazepam, have abuse potential and are commonly abused by patients with substance use disorders. When benzodiazepines must be used, then the longer-acting agents should be used. In addition, when longer-acting benzodiazepines are used in patients with a history of substance use disorders, records should carefully document the failure to respond to antidepressants and buspirone in patients who continue to be symptomatic.

Sleep disorders. Disturbances of sleep are common in patients with psychiatric disorders other than substance abuse, as well as in those with substance use disorders. The use of sedative-hypnotics should be avoided in dually diagnosed patients, especially those who are dependent on alcohol or opiates. Trazodone and zolpidem are two nonbenzodiazepines that are useful in the treatment of sleep disturbances in dually diagnosed patients.

Trazodone is the drug of choice for the treatment of insomnia in substance-abusing patients (Ware and Pittard 1990). Trazodone does not act on γ-aminobutyric acid (GABA) receptors and is not cross-tolerant with the benzodiazepines. Clinically, patients taking trazodone may complain of vivid dreams, sluggishness upon awakening, and grogginess in the morning. The well-known but low-frequency side effect of priapism should be explained to male patients when the medication is initiated. Some male patients may reject the use of trazodone, alleging priapism, in the hopes of getting a benzodiazepine substitute. However, a patient complaining of painful erections or spontaneous unwanted or unexpected erections should be instructed to discontinue trazodone. The soporific dose of trazodone is 50–150 mg per night.

Zolpidem is a nonbenzodiazepine sedative-hypnotic that acts at the GABA receptor. Although zolpidem is not thought to be as habituating as the benzodiazepines, care should be taken when prescribing this medication. Generally, zolpidem is recommended for short-term use; periods of less than 30 days are considered safe. We have used zolpidem sparingly in dually diagnosed patients. It is prescribed at 10 mg per night every other night. Patients are given limited prescriptions; no refills are permitted within the agreed-upon time period. Some dually diagnosed patients tolerate zolpidem well, whereas other patients complain that it produces a "high." One patient claimed that it increased his craving for cocaine. In short, zolpidem is a useful medication to provide acute relief from long periods of insomnia. However, unlike trazodone, zolpidem should be used with caution in dually diagnosed patients.

Opioid dependence. Opioid-dependent patients with comorbid psychiatric disorders other than substance abuse are best stabilized on methadone maintenance and then treated with the appropriate psychopharmacological agent that targets the symptoms of the non–substance abuse psychiatric condition. Hence, an opioid-dependent patient with psychosis would clearly benefit from both a neuroleptic and methadone maintenance. Methadone does not interfere with the functioning of either neuroleptics or antidepressants. In fact, Brizer et al. (1985) administered methadone to a small sample (four men and three women) of neuroleptic-resistant patients in a 3-week, single crossover study. The non–opioid-dependent patients received either 25 or 40 mg of methadone in addition to a neuroleptic and experienced a reduction in symptoms. Three patients showed clinical reductions in thought disorder, hallucinatory behavior, and paranoid ideation.

Levinson et al. (1995) warn that vulnerable patients withdrawing from methadone or other opioids may be at risk for the precipitation of a psychosis induced by the withdrawal process. Although withdrawal psychosis clearly occurs with low frequency, patients with a history of psychosis may be at risk. Thus, a patient on a methadone-tapering regimen who develops a "new" onset of psychosis should be treated with neuroleptics and a more careful history taken.

Nunes et al. (1991) reported that imipramine treatment was beneficial in 9 of 17 methadone-maintained patients with primary or chronic depression. The reported dosages of imipramine were within the normal therapeutic range. There did not appear to be any significant drug interactions between imipramine and methadone.

Since the Food and Drug Administration (FDA) approved the use of l-α-acetylmethadol (LAAM) in 1993, it is being adopted as an alternative to methadone maintenance. Although LAAM is similar to methadone, it is a long-acting compound that can be administered three times per week instead of the daily dosing associated with methadone. No difference is expected in LAAM's interactions with neuroleptics or antidepressants. Thus, dually diagnosed patients should benefit from this medication.

A third agent, buprenorphine, is being evaluated for approval by the FDA. Buprenorphine is different from both methadone and LAAM. Buprenorphine is a partial μ opiate agonist. Whereas at this point little is known about the use of LAAM in dually diagnosed patients, Bodkin et al. (1995) reported that buprenorphine may have an antidepressant effect. If further study supports this belief, then in depressed patients who tolerate or favor buprenorphine over methadone or LAAM, adjunctive effects might be achieved with the addition of an SSRI or a tricyclic antidepressant.

Opioid antagonists.   Naltrexone is a μ opiate receptor antagonist that was approved by the FDA in 1983 for use in opiate-addicted patients. Naltrexone binds to the μ opiate receptor and, to a lesser degree, the κ receptor. If a patient is pretreated, naltrexone's affinity for the μ opiate receptor blocks the effects of opioid drugs. Although the literature in this area is sparse, several reports suggest that an opioid antagonist like naltrexone could have a role in beneficially augmenting neuroleptic-stabilized schizophrenic patients (Berger et al. 1981; Rapaport et al. 1993; Watson et al. 1978).

The promise of naltrexone goes beyond neuroleptic augmentation. In 1995, the FDA approved its use in the treatment of alcoholism. Naltrexone supports abstinence, aids in decreasing craving and relapse, and decreases alcohol consumption. The utility of naltrexone for the spectrum of dually diagnosed patients has not been established. However, in the light of its side effect profile and the benefits already established, consideration should be given to using this agent in treating comorbid substance abuse and selected non–substance abuse psychiatric disorders when opiates or alcohol are involved.

Disulfiram—alcohol aversive.   Most clinicians are familiar with the use of disulfiram in the aversive treatment of an alcohol-abusing patient who is trying to avoid drinking. Ideally, within the context of dual diagnosis, disulfiram would be used to discourage or prevent patients from relapsing by producing the extremely uncomfortable reaction that is commonly known to the medical community. Disulfiram irreversibly inhibits the enzyme acetaldehyde dehydrogenase, permitting the accumulation of the toxic metabolite acetaldehyde when alcohol is consumed. The toxic metabolite quickly accumulates and produces well-known side effects. Side effects of disulfiram taken alone may include drowsiness, numbness in extremities, metallic taste, and allergic skin reaction.

Disulfiram plus alcohol may produce reactions. Even a small amount of alcohol taken while on disulfiram may produce redness of the face, throbbing in the head and neck, headache, breathing difficulties, stomach distress, vomiting, sweating, thirst, chest pain, fast heartbeat, faintness, marked uneasiness, weakness, sensation of surroundings revolving around you, blurred vision, and confusion. Rarely, in severe reactions, there may be a decrease in breathing, shock, acute heart failure, unconsciousness, convulsions, and death.

The disadvantage of disulfiram is that its utility as an oral medication is questionable. No reasonable evidence has been shown for the ability of disulfiram to increase patients' abstinence rates (Hughes and Cook 1997). In a review of 38 outcome studies, Hughes and Cook (1997) concluded that disulfiram may be helpful in reducing the quantity of alcohol consumed and reducing the number of drinking days.

An advantage of disulfiram is that it may be used—subject to the normal caveats—in dually diagnosed patients who can understand the inherent dangers of consuming even small quantities of alcohol while taking this medication. One group (Kofoed et al. 1986) reported that a small number of patients who had been stabilized on antipsychotics tolerated the use of disulfiram without untoward side effects, despite its postulated potential to exacerbate psychosis.

Nicotine dependence. The literature has now established a definite link between cigarette smoking and substance abuse. Many patients who abuse alcohol, stimulants, or opioids are also dependent on nicotine. It has also been established that depression, major depression, chronic schizophrenia, and anxiety disorders are associated with cigarette smoking (or, stated otherwise, nicotine dependence) (Glassman 1997). Among patients with schizophrenia, nicotine appears to be the most common substance of dependence (reviewed in Chapter 1).

Smoking cessation may precipitate depression in some individuals with a history of major depression, thereby producing a worse problem although the substance use disorder is "cured." Clearly, the concept of self-medication has currency in these individuals. Cornelius et al. (1997) conducted a double-blind, placebo-controlled trial of 25 smokers with diagnoses of major depressive disorder and alcohol dependence. The patients in the group taking fluoxetine experienced a significant within-group decrease in smoking during the study. Although the results were not statistically significant, the fluoxetine group smoked 27% fewer cigarettes than the placebo group and consumed four times less alcohol during the 12 weeks of the trial.

Although additional research is clearly needed, these preliminary findings indicate that fluoxetine has the potential for treating the smoking behaviors of depressed alcoholic smokers. Bupropion, on the other hand, has been approved by the FDA for use with depressed smokers. Research is needed to extend this approval to the use of bupropion for depressed smokers who also abuse alcohol, cocaine, or other substances.

Nicotine replacement therapies continue to be developed and disseminated. Currently, nicotine gum and nicotine patches are widely used. Conceptually, nicotine replacement is seen as mere substitution therapy, that is, as substituting pharmaceutical nicotine therapies for the more hazardous habits of smoking or tobacco chewing. However, it may be possible that the nicotine replacement therapy itself will play a role in the treatment of psychiatric disorders other than substance abuse or in substance use disorders other than nicotine use.

Special Diagnostic Issues in Dually Diagnosed Patients

In this section, we briefly discuss the three diagnostic areas of combat-related PTSD, sexual abuse, and eating disorders. Given that this is only a review article, insufficient attention can be given to these select issues. Yet no review of dual diagnosis is complete without some mention of them.

Combat-Related Posttraumatic Stress Disorder

Since the 1980s, much has been written about combat-related PTSD. Many authors have also addressed the relationship between combat-related PTSD and substance abuse. However, until the report of Bremner et al. (1996), little was written about the longitudinal characteristics of either PTSD symptoms or substance abuse in the military veteran population. Using the timeline follow-back technique, Bremner et al. (1996) evaluated a sample of 61 predominantly white ($n = 56$) Vietnam veterans with structured clinical interviews. In this group of veterans, three clusters of PTSD symptoms (intrusions, avoidance, and hyperarousal) were determined to develop within a few years after the Vietnam War. These symptoms soon became chronic. Subsequently, alcohol and substance abuse followed the increase in PTSD symptoms. In support of the self-medication hypothesis, Bremner et al. (1996) reported that veterans in the study considered the use of alcohol, heroin, marijuana, opiates, and benzodiazepines to be beneficial for their symptoms of PTSD. Their report also detailed the spectrum of pharmacological agents used by their sample for the treatment of PTSD: antidepressants, benzodiazepines, clonidine, buspirone, carbamazepine, valproic acid, propranolol, and neuroleptics. Oddly enough, although 58% of the sample received antidepressants during the course of their various treatments, more than half (57%) also received benzodiazepines. Among dually diagnosed patients, such liberal use of benzodiazepines is now discouraged.

Physical and Sexual Abuse

Increasing awareness of the impact of trauma on the lives of individuals has led to attempts to characterize the extent and the nature of that trauma. Contemporary physical and sexual abuse are associated with PTSD. Furthermore, the use of substances of abuse by victims of physical and sexual abuse—domestic violence, rape, or assault—has been established.

In recent years attempts have been made to characterize the occurrence of physical and sexual abuse and associated psychiatric disorders among populations of patients in substance abuse treatment (Mindle et al. 1995). It is critical for clinicians to realize that the overall prevalence of childhood abuse may be quite high in people who present for substance abuse treatment. Mindle et al. (1995) reported that, among a population of alcoholic inpatients, 59% of the women and 30% of the men reported childhood abuse. However, almost half (49%) of the women and 12% of the men reported sexual abuse (with or without physical abuse). Because there are high rates of adult psychiatric symptoms among victims of childhood abuse, especially sexual abuse, it is important for clinicians to assess any patient presenting with psychiatric symptoms for past childhood physical or sexual abuse (Rosenberg et al. 1996). Furthermore, it is important for those who are treating patients presenting for substance abuse to likewise assess for childhood trauma. Rosenberg et al. (1996) contend that cognitive-behavioral treatment approaches to women with PTSD offer promise. Clearly, treatment strategies for both women and men who have been subjected to either childhood or adult physical or sexual trauma need to be further developed and employed.

Eating Disorders

Studies indicate that the rate of substance abuse is elevated among women with eating disorders. However, it does not appear that the rate of anorexia is elevated among alcoholic patients after controlling for other disorders. Furthermore, although the rate of bulimia is elevated, it is not remarkably so. Finally, both anorexia and bulimia appear to be relatively rare among men and women who present for substance abuse treatment (Schuckit et al. 1996).

Integration of Treatment Modalities in Dually Diagnosed Patients

Nonpharmacological treatments of dually diagnosed patients should encompass the use of a spectrum of services in order to meet patients' needs. Higher-functioning dually diagnosed patients require different interventions than do more severely ill patients. Given the brevity of this chapter, we do not explore the separate psychotherapeutic techniques available for the treatment of higher-functioning patients. We refer to higher functioning in areas such as: interpersonal relationships, housing, education, employment, income, and family relationships. Although these areas of functioning can be impaired in a patient with any type of psychiatric disorder, whether substance use or non-substance use, they are certainly more impaired in those patients who are commonly served by the public mental health delivery system. Clinicians should bear in mind the caveat that, regardless of the service delivery system that is available and the constellation of treatments employed, communication between service providers is critical so that providers of substance abuse treatment and non–substance abuse treatment are not operating at loggerheads.

For patients whose psychiatric problems cause severe impairment in levels of functioning, a more integrated treatment approach is warranted. Current treatment approaches for dually diagnosed patients dictate that intensive and specific treatments for both illnesses be provided concomitantly. Tsuang et al. (1997) described a dual diagnosis program that included pharmacotherapy, psychoeducation, behavioral interventions, skills training, and case management. Substance abuse treatment revolved around a focus of harm reduction and relapse prevention.

Ideally, a "one-stop shop" approach should be employed to prevent patients from falling between the cracks created by the separation of substance abuse and non–substance abuse mental health services (Drake 1996; Drake et al. 1997). In addition to medication, the provision of a full spectrum of services also benefits the larger community through decreases in emergency room visits, hospitalization, drug or alcohol use, and homelessness and other social problems. S. Brady et al. (1996) stress that to be effective, treatment programs should not have rigid policies that mandate clients to be clean and sober before receiving non–substance use mental health services or to be otherwise psychiatrically stable prior to receiving substance abuse services.

A key clinical issue in the provision of treatment for dually diagnosed patients is the willingness and motivation of staff to work with complex patients. Ridgely and Jerrell (1996) provided qualitative data from an analysis of three interventions for sub-stance abuse treatment of severely mentally ill patients. They concluded that successful programs have the following components:

- Sufficient time set aside to work with patients
- Small staff caseloads
- Clinical management and supervisory support for staff
- Teams to minimize staff burnout
- Professional latitude and discretion to make adjustments in interventions

From a substance abuse perspective, Ridgely and Jerrell (1996) found the following three models to be promising for dually diagnosed patients:

1. Twelve-step social recovery
2. Behavioral skills training
3. Intensive case management

From the perspective of diagnosing psychiatric disorders other than substance abuse, behavioral skills training and intensive case management would certainly address the unique needs of severely mentally ill patients. Thus, a comprehensive approach to the patient's needs can be achieved.

Summary

The phenomenon of dual diagnosis remains complex. The developments described in this chapter represent only a portion of the evolving base of knowledge on dual diagnosis. The clinician's ability to manage dually diagnosed patients is obviously enhanced by having an appropriate suspicion of the use of alcohol or drugs in patients presenting with a psychiatric disorder other than substance abuse. Alternatively, it is equally important to explore the possibility of a comorbid non–substance abuse psychiatric disorder in patients presenting for substance abuse treatment.

In recent years, the label *substance use disorder* has become associated with the loss of safety-sensitive employment, social security benefits, and worker's compensation benefits. Thus, the clinician can provide patients with appropriate clinical care by attempting to accurately diagnose the patient's condition. After an accurate diagnosis has been established, the use of an appropriate pharmacological agent may be critical to reduce the patient's symptoms. At this point, with the exception of opioid replacement therapy, the most substantial pharmacological intervention can be made in the area of non–substance use psychiatric symptoms. Thus, careful attention to the selection of the appropriate pharmacological agent and to medication compliance is warranted. In the end, psychosocial interventions, in conjunction with psychopharmacology, will undoubtedly produce the best improvement in patient symptoms.

Ongoing research, both basic and clinical, is needed in order to gain a better understanding of the context and solutions of dual diagnosis. With changes in service delivery systems, both for the treatment of substance use disorders and non–substance use psychiatric disorders, it is important for resources to be allocated for more sophisticated studies in epidemiology, health services, medication, and psychosocial interventions.

References

American Psychiatric Association: Diagnostic and Statistical Manual of Mental Disorders, 4th Edition. Washington, DC, American Psychiatric Association, 1994

Appleby L, Dyson V, Altman E, et al: Assessing substance use in multiproblem patients: reliability and validity of the Addiction Severity Index in a mental hospital population. J Nerv Ment Dis 185(3):159–165, 1997

Berger PA, Watson SJ, Akil H, et al: The effects of naloxone in chronic schizophrenia. Am J Psychiatry 138(7):913–918, 1981

Berger SP, Hall S, Mickalian JD, et al: Haloperidol antagonism of cue-elicited cocaine craving. Lancet 347:504–508, 1996

Bersoff DN, Glass DJ, Blain N: Legal issues in the assessment and treatment of individuals with dual diagnoses. J Consult Clin Psychol 62(1):55–62, 1994

Bodkin JA, Zornberg GL, Lukas SE, et al: Buprenorphine treatment of refractory depression. J Clin Psychopharmacol 15(1):49–57, 1995

Boyd MR, Hauenstein EJ: Psychiatric assessment and confirmation of dual disorders in rural substance abusing women. Arch Psychiatr Nurs 11(2):74–81, 1997

Brady KT, Sonne SC, Anton R, et al: Valproate in the treatment of acute bipolar affective episodes complicated by substance abuse: a pilot study. J Clin Psychiatry 56:118–121, 1995

Brady S, Hiam CM, Saemann R, et al: Dual diagnosis: a treatment model for substance abuse and major mental illness. Community Ment Health J 32(6):573–578, 1996

Bremner JD, Southwick SM, Darnell A, et al: Chronic PTSD in Vietnam combat veterans: course of illness and substance abuse. Am J Psychiatry 153(3):369–375, 1996

Brizer DA, Hartman N, Seeney J, et al: Effect of methadone plus neuroleptics on treatment-resistant chronic paranoid schizophrenia. Am J Psychiatry 142:1106–1107, 1985

Brooner RK, King VL, Kidorf M, et al: Psychiatric and substance use comorbidity among treatment-seeking opioid abusers. Arch Gen Psychiatry 54:71–80, 1997

Buydens-Branchey L, Branchey M, Fergeson P, et al: Craving for cocaine in addicted users: role of serotonergic mechanisms. Am J Addictions 6(1):65–73, 1997

Carey KB: Substance use reduction in the context of outpatient psychiatric treatment: a collaborative, motivational, harm reduction approach. Community Ment Health J 32(3):291–306, 1996

Carey KB, Cocco KM, Simons JS: Concurrent validity of clinicians' ratings of substance abuse among psychiatric outpatients. Psychiatric Services 47(8):842–847, 1996

Casey DE: The relationship of pharmacology to side effects. J Clin Psychiatry 58(suppl 10):55–62, 1997

Castaneda R, Sussaman N, Westreich L, et al: A review of the effects of moderate alcohol intake on the treatment of anxiety and mood disorders. J Clin Psychiatry 57(5):207–212, 1996

Claassen C, Gilfillan S, Orsulak P, et al: Substance use among patients with a psychotic disorder in a psychiatric emergency room. Psychiatric Services 48(3):353–358, 1997

Cornelius JR, Salloum IM, Ehler JG, et al: Double-blind fluoxetine in depressed alcoholic smokers. Psychopharmacol Bull 33(1):165–170, 1997

Derogatis LR: Administration, Scoring, and Procedures Manual, II. Baltimore, MD, Clinical Psychometric Research, 1983

Drake RE: Substance use reduction among patients with severe mental illness. Community Ment Health J 32(3):311–314, 1996

Drake RE, Yovetich NA, Rebout RR, et al: Integrated treatment for dually diagnosed homeless adults. J Nerv Ment Dis 185:298–305, 1997

Gastfriend DR: Pharmacological treatments for psychiatric symptoms in addiction populations, in The Principles and Practice of Addictions in Psychiatry. Edited by Miller NS. Philadelphia, PA, WB Saunders, 1997, pp 486–495

Glassman AH: Cigarette smoking and its comorbidity. NIDA Research Monograph No 172. NIH Publ No 97-4172. Washington, DC, National Institutes of Health, 1997, pp 52–60

Goldfinger SM, Schutt RK, Seidman LJ, et al: Self-report and observer measures of substance abuse among homeless mentally ill persons in the cross-section and over time. J Nerv Ment Dis 184(11):667–672, 1996

Gorelick DA, Paredes A: Effect of fluoxetine on alcohol consumption in male alcoholics. Alcohol Clin Exp Res 16(2):261–265, 1992

Grabowsky J, Rhoades H, Elf R, et al: Fluoxetine is ineffective for treatment of cocaine dependence or concurrent opiate and cocaine dependence: two placebo controlled double-blind trials. J Clin Psychopharmacol 15:163–174, 1995

Grady TA, Broocks A, Canter SK, et al: Biological and behavioral responses to D-amphetamine, alone and in combination with the serotonin-3 receptor antagonist ondansetron, in healthy volunteers. Psychiatry Res 64(1):1–10, 1996

Halikas JA, Croby RD, Pearson VL, et al: A randomized double-blind study of carbamazepine in the treatment of cocaine abuse. Clin Pharmacol Ther 62(1):89–105, 1997

Hasin DS, Trautman KD, Miele GM, et al: Psychiatric research interview for substance and mental disorders (PRISM): reliability for substance abusers. Am J Psychiatry 153(9):1195–1201, 1996

Helzer JE, Pryzbeck TR: The co-occurrence of alcoholism with other psychiatric disorders in the general population and its impact on treatment. J Stud Alcohol 49(3):219–224, 1988

Hodgins DC, El-Guebaly N: More data on the Addiction Severity Index: reliability and validity with the mentally ill substance abuser. J Nerv Ment Dis 180:197–201, 1992

Hughes JC, Cook CC: The efficacy of disulfiram: a review of outcome studies. Addiction 92(4):381–395, 1997

Janssen E: A self psychological approach to treating the mentally ill, chemical abusing and addicted (MICAA) patient. Arch Psychiatr Nurs 8(6):381–389, 1994

Keller MB, Lavori PW, Coryell W, et al: Differential outcome of pure manic, mixed/cycling, and pure depressive episodes in patients with bipolar illness. JAMA 255:3138–3142, 1986

Kofoed L, Kania J, Walsh T, et al: Outpatient treatment of patients with substance abuse and coexisting psychiatric disorders. Am J Psychiatry 143(7):867–872, 1986

Kranzler HR, Burleson JA, Del Boca FK, et al: Buspirone treatment of anxious alcoholics: a placebo-controlled trial. Arch Gen Psychiatry 51(9):720–731, 1994

Kranzler HR, Burleson JA, Brown J, et al: Fluoxetine treatment seems to reduce the beneficial effects of cognitive-behavioral therapy in type B alcoholics. Alcohol Clin Exp Res 20(9):1534–1541, 1996

Levinson I, Galynker II, Rosenthal RN: Methadone withdrawal psychosis. J Clin Psychiatry 56(2):73–76, 1995

Marcus P, Snyder R: Reduction of comorbid substance abuse with clozapine. Am J Psychiatry 152:6, 1995

Mason BJ, Kocsis JH, Ritvo EC, et al: A double-blind, placebo-controlled trial of desipramine for primary alcohol dependence stratified on the presence or absence of major depression. JAMA 275(10):761–767, 1996

McGrath PJ, Nunes EV, Stewart JW, et al: Imipramine treatment of alcoholics with primary depression: a placebo-controlled clinical trial. Arch Gen Psychiatry 53(3):232–240, 1996

McLellan AT, Kushner H, Metzger D, et al: The fifth edition of the Addiction Severity Index. J Subst Abuse Treat 9:199–213, 1992

Mindle M, Windle RC, Scheidt DM, et al: Physical and sexual abuse and associated mental disorders among alcoholic inpatients. Am J Psychiatry 152:1322–1328, 1995

Mueller TI, Goldenberg IM, Gordon AL, et al: Benzodiazepine use in anxiety disordered patients with and without a history of alcoholism. J Clin Psychiatry 57(2):83–89, 1996

National Institute on Drug Abuse: Epidemiologic Trends in Drug Abuse, Vol I: Highlights and Executive Summary. NIH Publ No 96-4126. Bethesda, MD, National Institutes of Health, 1996

Nunes EV, Quitkin FM, Brady R, et al: Imipramine treatment of methadone maintenance patients with affective disorder and illicit drug use. Am J Psychiatry 148(5):667–669, 1991

Nunes EV, McGrath PJ, Quitkin FM, et al: Imipramine treatment of alcoholism with comorbid depression. Am J Psychiatry 150:963–965, 1993

O'Brien CP: Recent developments in the pharmacology of substance abuse. J Consult Clin Psychol 64(4):677–686, 1996

Owen RR, Fischer EP, Booth BM, et al: Medication noncompliance and substance abuse among patients with schizophrenia. Psychiatric Services 47(8):853–858, 1996

Pechter BM, Janicak PG, Davis JM: Psychopharmacotherapy for the dually diagnosed: novel approaches, in The Principles and Practice of Addictions in Psychiatry. Edited by Miller NS. Philadelphia, PA, WB Saunders, 1997, pp 521–531

Rapaport MH, Wolkowitz O, Kelsoe JR, et al: Beneficial effects of nalmefene augmentation in neuroleptic-stabilized schizophrenic patients. Neuropsychopharmacology 9(2):111–115, 1993

Regier DA, Framer ME, Rae DS, et al: Comorbidity of mental disorders with alcohol and other drug abuse: results from the Epidemiologic Catchment Area (ECA) Study. JAMA 264(19):2511–2518, 1990

Ridgely MS, Jerrell JM: Analysis of three interventions for substance abuse treatment of severely mentally ill people. Community Ment Health J 32(6):561–572, 1996

Rosenberg SD, Drake RE, Mueser K: New directions for treatment research on sequelae of sexual abuse in persons with severe mental illness. Community Ment Health J 32:387–400, 1996

Schuckit MA, Tipp JE, Anthenelli RM, et al: Anorexia nervosa and bulimia nervosa in alcohol-dependent men and women and their relatives. Am J Psychiatry 153:74–82, 1996

Self DW, Banhart WJ, Lehman DA: Opposite modulation of cocaine-seeking behavior by D_1 and D_2-like dopamine receptor agonists. Science 27:1586–1589, 1996

Sonne SC, Brady KT, Morton WA: Substance abuse and bipolar affective disorder. J Nerv Ment Dis 182:349–352, 1994

Spitzer RL, Williams JB, Gibbon M, et al: Structured Clinical Interview for DSM-III-R, Patient Version (SCID-P). New York, New York State Psychiatric Institute, Biometrics Research, 1990

Tsuang JW, Ho AP, Eckman TA, et al: Dual diagnosis treatment for patients with schizophrenia who are substance dependent. Psychiatric Services 48(7):887–889, 1997

Ware JC, Pittard JT: Increased deep sleep after trazodone use: a double-blind placebo-controlled study in healthy young adults. J Clin Psychiatry 51(suppl 9):18–22, 1990

Watson SJ, Berger PA, Akil H, et al: Effects of naloxone on schizophrenia: reduction in hallucinations in a subpopulation of subjects. Science 201:73–76, 1978

Wilkins J: Pharmacotherapy of schizophrenia patients with comorbid substance abuse. Schizophr Bull 23(2):215–228, 1997

Yovell Y: Clozapine reverses cocaine craving in a treatment-resistant mentally ill chemical abuser: a case report and a hypothesis. J Nerv Ment Dis 182(10):591–592, 1994

Ziedonis DM, Kosten TR: Pharmacotherapy improves treatment outcome in depressed cocaine addicts. J Psychoactive Drugs 23:417–425, 1991

Zinermon v Burch, 494 U.S. 113 (1990)

Afterword

Elinore F. McCance-Katz, M.D., Ph.D., and
Thomas R. Kosten, M.D.

The chapters in this monograph should have provided the clinician with an overview of important topics in addictions at the present time and the probable directions of the field in the next few years.

In Chapter 1, Ziedonis and colleagues underscore the magnitude of the problem of nicotine dependence. Their review serves as a reminder to psychiatry that nicotine dependence is a serious disorder with medical and psychological sequelae that must be addressed in the treatment of patients presenting for psychiatric or substance abuse treatment. The issue of cigarette smoking has been largely ignored by mental health professionals to date, but the impact of this problem on patients' overall physical health, psychological states, and psychotropic medication levels can have great importance to response to treatment. Recent research demonstrating nicotine's common neurobiological pathways with other drugs of abuse emphasizes its potential as a "gateway" drug but also presents intriguing possibilities for the development of treatments that simultaneously target multiple substance use disorders. Ongoing research is better defining optimal treatment regimens and matching patients to treatments of optimal duration.

The treatment of substance-related disorders has been based mostly on experiences with males. The optimal treatment modalities for women with substance abuse disorders remain the focus of research studies. These studies examine how to provide for the specialized needs of women in treatment and how to understand the impact of the biological differences between men and women in their responses to drugs and alcohol. In Chapter 2, Myroslava Romach and Edward Sellers provide an excellent review of the current state of knowledge about alcohol abuse in women. In Chapter 3, Susan Stine points out the difficulties in treating women who are opioid-dependent. Together these authors show the need for new research on gender-related issues in substance abuse treatment.

Opioid dependence treatment options are quickly expanding with the advent of new pharmacotherapies that appear to have efficacies similar to those of methadone maintenance but that broaden the treatment settings available to opioid-dependent patients. Research is now addressing issues about whether these new agents confer additional advantages. Such advantages include a reduction of cocaine or other substance use, a problem shown to be quite prevalent in heroin users and methadone-maintained patients, and whether a transition to drug-free treatment might be facilitated by nonmethadone maintenance agents after a circumscribed period of maintenance treatment. Finally, what drug combinations are optimal for opioid-dependent patients with other medical illnesses such as HIV disease or hepatitis will be of great assistance to the practicing clinician.

The increasing contribution of drug abusers to the ranks of those with HIV disease is an unfortunate reality that must be addressed by both psychiatric and medical providers. In Chapter 4, Robert Cabaj provides a stark overview of the magnitude and complexity of the problem represented by substance abusers with HIV disease. In his chapter, we also learn about the nuances of treatment of this impaired population. Questions remain regarding optimal treatment settings, pharmacotherapy regimens for HIV disease and psychiatric or substance-related disorders, how to address issues of substance abuse and HIV disease simultaneously, and what methods will impart necessary information about healthier lifestyles to patients in a way that they can comprehend and put into practice.

Advances in our understanding of dually diagnosed patients have clearly been made in recent years and are highlighted in Chapter 5 by Westley Clark and Terry McClanahan. However, much remains to be elucidated by further research in regard to the neurobiology and pathophysiology of substance-related disorders that have presentations similar to psychiatric disorders. An understanding of the relationship between these disorders could provide important clues to the development of new and effective treatment modalities. Clark and McClanahan also discuss considerations that are important to providing optimal care to dually diagnosed patients—care that considers the treatment modalities shown to be most effective to date as well as staff needs in coping with this demanding and complex population.

The chapters in this monograph highlight a number of important and timely topics in addiction medicine that are important to the practicing clinician. These works cover issues ranging from epidemiology to treatment of these disorders. The pharmacological and psychological interventions presented can provide the foundation for improved treatments and preventive interventions in these addicted populations of patients.

Index

*Page numbers printed in **boldface** type refer to tables or figures.*

Cognitive effects
  of alcohol, 43, **44–47**
    combined with disulfiram,
      172
  of neuroleptics, 162
Coma, opioid-induced, 77
Combat-related posttraumatic
    stress disorder, 174
"Coming out," 140
Compliance with treatment
  of dually diagnosed patients,
    161–162
  of HIV-infected substance
    abusers, 94–95, 127–128
Computerized tomography, 41
Concentration problems, 8
Confusion, drug-induced
  benzodiazepines, 131
  disulfiram combined with
    alcohol, 172
Contemplation Ladder, 9
Coronary artery disease, 43
Cortisol, 164
Coughing
  associated with nicotine
    withdrawal, 8
  induced by nicotine nasal
    spray, 18
Counseling, as adjunct to
    methadone maintenance
    treatment, 89–90
Crack cocaine, 117, 139
"Crank," 115
Craving
  for cocaine, 164, 169
  for nicotine, 8
  for opioids, 77, 78, 84
Criminal behavior
  opiate dependence and, 75
  of persons in methadone
    maintenance programs,
      86, 88, 89

"Crystal," 115
Cyclic adenosine
    monophosphate (cAMP), 80
Cytochrome P450 enzymes
  metabolism of ethanol by,
    38, 39
  metabolism of protease
    inhibitors by, 96

Day treatment programs for
    methadone-maintained
    patients, 90–91
Defense mechanisms, 120
Dehydroepiandrosterone, 42
Delavirdine, 95
Delirium, 160
  HIV infection and, 134
  precipitated by substance
    withdrawal
    benzodiazepines, 132
    central nervous system
      depressants, 126
Delirium tremens, 132
Dementia, HIV, 134, 136
Demoralization, 132
Denial, 120, 136
Dependent personality disorder,
    154
Depression, 159
  alcohol dependence and, 36,
    51–54
    antidepressant therapy
      and, 53–54
    self-medication hypothesis
      of, 48–49, 52
    in women, 52–53
  estrogen and, 53
  in HIV-infected substance
    abusers, 132–134
  insomnia due to, 132
  nicotine dependence and,
    8, 24–25

Drug interactions
with methadone, 87, 95, 96,
127, 161, 170
with monoamine oxidase
inhibitors, 133
with nicotine, 13, **13**
with protease inhibitors, 96
Drug-seeking behavior, 77, 85
Dry mouth, bupropion-induced,
19
Dual diagnosis, 151–178, 184–185
assessment, evaluation, and
diagnosis of, 154–157
clinical presentations of
persons with, 160
clusters of comorbidity,
155–156
complexity of, 177
contemporary assessment and
legal rights of persons
with, 157–159, 177–178
definition of, 151
differentiating effects of
psychoactive substances
from symptoms of
psychiatric disorder, 151
epidemiology of, 152–154
prevalence of, 155
reliability of self-reports of
substance abuse, 156
traditional schools of thought
regarding, 156
Dual diagnosis treatment,
159–178
inefficiency of programs for,
151–152
integration of, 175–177
for patients with combat-
related posttraumatic
stress disorder, 174
for patients with eating
disorders, 175

psychopharmacotherapeutics,
159–173
for anxiety disorders,
167–168
for bipolar affective
episodes, 164–165
choice of medications, 161
decision to use
medications, 160
disulfiram, 171–172
for major depression,
166–167
medication
noncompliance,
161–162
neurobiology and,
160–161
neuroleptics, 162–164
for nicotine dependence,
172–173
opioid antagonists, 171
for opioid dependence,
169–171
for sleep disorders, 169
for victims of physical and
sexual abuse, 174–175
Due process rights, 157–158
Dynorphin, 79
Dysphoria
during nicotine withdrawal, 8
premenstrual, 55
Dysthymic disorder
smoking and, 25
substance-induced, 154

Eating disorders, 175
ECA. *See* Epidemiologic
Catchment Area study
"Ecstasy," 117
Electroencephalography during
nicotine withdrawal, 8
Employment counseling, 90

5-HT. *See* Serotonin
Human immunodeficiency virus
(HIV) infection and
substance abuse, 94–96,
113–144, 184
assessment of, 121–124
bacterial infections and, 97
case management for,
128–129
children of persons with,
142–143
drugs and sexual activity and,
115–116, 120
epidemiology of, 114–115
injection drug use and, 94, 95,
114–116, 120
losses associated with, 138
opiate dependence and,
75, 94–96
socioeconomic status and,
117–118
specific drugs abused in,
116–117
standards of care for, 125
stigma and prejudice about,
113–114, 121–122
tuberculosis and, 94, 97
among women, 116, 142
Human immunodeficiency virus
(HIV) infection and
substance abuse treatment,
118–144
adherence and
noncompliance with,
94–95, 127–128
avoiding provider burnout in,
144
barriers to, 125
challenges in, 143
educational efforts and,
121, 129–130
goal of, 118–119

harm reduction models of,
118–119, 124–125, 144
inpatient, 126
for intoxicated patients,
125–126
matching treatment with
patient, 121
mental health interventions,
94, 130–139, 143–144
pharmacotherapy for
anxiety, 131–132
pharmacotherapy for
depression, 132–134
pharmacotherapy for
insomnia, 132
pharmacotherapy for
psychosis, 134
provider's attitudes and,
134–135
psychotherapy, 137–139
for suicidality, 135–137
targeting to specific
populations, 130
prevention strategies,
129–130, 144
relapse prevention model for,
125, 138, 144
residential programs for, 119
seeking and entering, 119–121
for special populations,
139–143
gay and bisexual men,
139–141
people of color, 143
women and children,
142–143
youth, 142
toxicities of drug therapy for,
95–96
twelve-step programs for, 119
understanding options for,
119

LC (Locus ceruleus), 80–81
Legal issues, 157–159
Lesbians, 116, 129, 130, 139, 141
  adolescent, 142
Liberty principle, 157
Lipid abnormalities,
  ritonavir-induced, 95
Lithium
  for alcohol dependence, 59, **60**
  for comorbid substance abuse
    and bipolar disorder, 165
Liver disease
  drug-induced, 97
    alcohol, 41, 42, 96
    antiretroviral agents, 95
    neuroleptics, 162
    valproate, 165
  effect on methadone
    metabolism, 87
  injection drug use and, 96–97
  psychiatric disorders and, 98
  treating opioid dependence in
    patients with, 87, 96–97
Locus ceruleus (LC), 80–81
Lorazepam, **13**
  use in dually diagnosed
    patients, 161
  for withdrawal from central
    nervous system
    depressants, 126
LSD (Lysergic acid
  diethylamide), 117
Luteinizing hormone, 42
Lysergic acid diethylamide
  (LSD), 117

Mania
  lithium for, 165
  opiate dependence and, 98
  treating substance abuse and,
    164–165
  valproate for, 164–165

Marijuana use, 152, 163, 174
  comorbid with opioid
    dependence, 154
  HIV infection and, 115, 116
MAST (Michigan Alcohol
  Screening Test), 62
MDMA (3,4-Methylenedioxy-
  methamphetamine), 117
Mecamylamine for smoking
  cessation, 16
  combining with nicotine
    transdermal patch, 22–23
Medically ill patients
  HIV infection, 94–96, 113–144
  methadone metabolism in, 87
  treating opiate dependence in,
    94–97, 184
Meditation, 131
Memory effects of nicotine, 5
Memory impairment, 160
  benzodiazepine-induced, 131
Menstrual cycle
  alcohol effects during, 55–56
  sex hormone effects, 41–42
    effect on ethanol kinetics,
      39–40
    hepatic dysfunction and, 42
Meperidine, 82
Metabolic rate
  during nicotine withdrawal, 8
  after opiate detoxification, 85
Methadone
  for detoxification, 83, 127
  drug interactions with, 87, 95,
    96, 127, 161, 170
  effect on cocaine-induced
    euphoria, 92
  factors affecting metabolism
    of, 87
  overdose of, 82
  time to onset of withdrawal
    from, 77

Psychosocial treatments
for HIV-infected persons, 94
for opiate dependence, 75,
88–91
for smoking cessation, 12, **12,**
14–16
Psychotherapy
for depression, 133
for dually diagnosed patients,
175–177
for HIV-infected substance
abusers, 121, 137–139
PTSD. *See* Posttraumatic stress
disorder
Public housing benefits, 159
Pulmonary edema, 82
Pulse Check, 75
Pupillary contraction, 77, 103
Pupillary dilation, 77

Rape victims, 174
Rational emotive therapy, 26
Reason for Quitting Scale, 9
Reimbursement for smoking
cessation treatment, 3, 11
Relapse prevention model
for HIV-infected substance
abusers, 125, 138, 144
for opiate-dependent persons,
78
Relapses, 78, 84, 120, 121
Relaxation therapy, 26
Renal disease, 87
Resources on smoking cessation,
2–3, 11
Respiratory depression,
opioid-induced, 77
naloxone reversal of, 82
Restlessness during substance
withdrawal
nicotine, 8
opiates, 77

Reverse transcriptase inhibitors,
95
Rhinorrhea
induced by nicotine nasal
spray, 18
during opioid withdrawal,
78
Rifabutin, interaction with
methadone, 127
Rifampin, 97
interaction with methadone,
87, 127
Risperidone, 162
Ritanserin for alcohol
dependence, 58, 59, **60**
Ritonavir, 95–96

Sadness, 132
Safer-sex practices, 114–116, 129
Saquinavir, 95–96
Schizophrenia, 134, 152, 159
atypical neuroleptics for, 162
P50 auditory-evoked
responses in, 27
substance abuse and, 152, 162
cocaine, 163
nicotine, 20, 26–27
opiates, 98, 153
pharmacotherapy for,
163
self-medication hypothesis
of, 162–163
Schizophreniform disorders,
152
SCID. *See* Structured Clinical
Interview for DSM-III-R or
DSM-IV
SCID-P. *See* Structured Clinical
Interview for DSM-IV—
Patient Version
SCL-90-R. *See* Symptom
Checklist

DATE DUE